TRUE BRAIN FITNESS

Preventing Brain Aging *through* Body Movement

DR. AIHAN KUHN

iUniverse, Inc.
New York   Bloomington

True Brain Fitness
Preventing Brain Aging through Body Movement

iUniverse books may be ordered through booksellers or by contacting:

iUniverse
1663 Liberty Drive
Bloomington, IN 47403
www.iuniverse.com
1-800-Authors (1-800-288-4677)

ISBN: 978-1-4502-6654-3 (sc)
ISBN: 978-1-4502-6656-7 (dj)
ISBN: 978-1-4502-6655-0 (ebook)

Printed in the United States of America

iUniverse rev. date: 11/30/2010

Publisher's Note

This book is intended to assist people concerned about brain aging and memory loss and also to help tai chi chuan students to understand the true nature of tai chi and qigong practice, and to help them to achieve the maximum benefits from learning tai chi, especially its anti-aging benefits. This book is not intended to treat any illness, nor as a substitute for medicine or treatment by a physician. Please ask your healthcare provider if you have any medical concerns.

Books, DVDs, workshops, and appointments are available at
Chinese Medicine for Health
1564A Washington Street
Holliston, MA 01746

To find out more or sign up for our newsletter,
please call us at (508) 429–3895
or visit www.ChineseMedicineforHealth.com

Other Books by Aihan Kuhn:

Natural Healing with Qigong

Simple Chinese Medicine

Tai Chi for Depression

With love and thanks to my many helpers.

Acknowledgments

It took a great deal of time and effort to figure out how to say things right, how to put the language into the right order and make good sentences. In Chinese, we speak and write in the opposite order from English; so we say, "English speaks opposite." On the other hand, an English speaker could say we speak in the opposite order. I have improved a great deal in my speaking and my writing, but I am still learning every day, every month, and every year. To finish this book, I still needed a lot of help. Luckily, I have many very good people around me, giving me support, not only with my language, but also with many other aspects of my work and my life. Therefore, I would like to take this opportunity to thank all the people who have helped me, who reviewed this book, who made many corrections, and who gave me a great deal of encouragement.

A tai chi book is not too hard for me to write, because I have been teaching it for over twenty years. To clearly describe the benefits to our brains, however, is much more complicated. I've done a lot of research, reading, and studying, trying to identify the connections between Eastern and Western science, and to explain why tai chi is so beneficial. I would like to thank Marie Murphy and Michele Talabach, who have been teaching young people with learning disabilities and behavior problems, and providing counseling at the college level for many years. I also would like to thank Pam Formosa, who has been teaching "Brain Gym" for many years, and told me "there are many similarities between Brain Gym, qigong, and tai chi." Her words helped to convince me that I was on the right track. I would like to thank my good friend Mary Beth Kahler, who helped me with my language any time I needed it.

I am very thankful to my husband, Gerry Kuhn, always the first person to read my drafts and do the first round of editing. I would like to thank my son, Peter Kuhn, who has helped me with both my work *and* my language. I would also like to thank Ron Weinberg, who is always watching over me and helping me on my path to success.

Thanks go to our tai chi instructors and assistant instructors, Jeanne Donnelly, Joe Foley, Shawn Armacost, Alon Harpaz, and Vic Cevoli. Even though some of them have moved away, their feedback has always helped me in both tai chi language and tai chi data building.

Thank you to everyone who read and appreciated my first book, *Natural*

Healing with Qigong, and my second book, *Simple Chinese Medicine*, which has been honored as a finalist in the Health: Alternative Medicine category of the National Best Books 2009 awards, sponsored by *USA Book News*. Thanks especially to those readers who gave me so much positive feedback on Amazon. You gave me the encouragement to continue writing and exploring human energy science, preventive medicine, and natural healing.

I always tell myself I am grateful, and I am very thankful for all the help I receive.

Dr. Aihan Kuhn
March 2010

Contents

Preface

I studied conventional Western medicine in medical school in China from 1977 to 1982. Much of the information in this book is based on general information I learned in medical school blended together with practical knowledge I gathered from my natural healing practice. Information used in this book also comes from other reputable sources. I have done my best to synthesize my tai chi experience with my medical and scientific knowledge.

When I was young, I used to wonder why the tai chi and qigong masters were so smart, so healthy, so calm, and so cool. When I started to learn tai chi, I just wanted to be like them. In the first several years, I did not feel any dramatic difference in those areas, but I did feel good overall, in health and wellbeing. Now I have been teaching and practicing for a long time, and as the years have gone by, I have started to see the difference. I have started to see myself as a different person, as a master of my own life.

I used to have a poor memory, perhaps from my poor genes, because my parents had poor health. My mother and her family had arthritis, and my father had tuberculosis when he was nine years old. In his middle age, he had chronic bronchitis and asthma, which often turned to pneumonia. My poor memory showed in school—especially medical school. It took me twice as long to learn, sometimes three times as long to memorize the coursework as it took my classmates.

In Chinese medicine, the brain is related to *kidney* energy. If you have poor kidney energy (and I was apparently born this way), you will have memory issues, arthritis issues, hair issues, teeth issues, and bone issues. Actually, I have all of these. My saving grace is that I am a tai chi and qigong practitioner. Though I have many issues, I don't have too many symptoms that affect my life, my work, or my career. The first thing I have noticed is my memory has not diminished. This is odd, because it should be worsening with age. But, it is almost the same as always. In some ways, it is even better than before.

The next thing I noticed is my learning ability. I wasn't born smart: I could never picture myself using a computer before. I used to get lost when driving somewhere, even though I had been there before. I had a hard time reading a map; it was just too confusing. I remember one time when I finished teaching a class at a new place at night; I drove thirty miles in the wrong direction while trying to get home. I ended up calling the police department to have a policeman guide me back to the highway, so that I could get home. By the time I got home, it was almost midnight. And I would never have thought that I could speak in public. I could barely make it though talks with groups of friends when I was younger. Here, it's even worse; living in a different country and struggling with English, how could I give public speeches? Now in contrast, I do use a computer everyday, and I often get compliments from my computer-geek husband. I make fewer wrong turns when I go to new places, and I can use a map wisely. I give speeches in many places, with trainings, lectures, workshops, and teaching on a regular basis. I attribute all of these improvements to my tai chi and qigong practice and teaching.

I share this with you because I believe that anyone who is willing to change and do things for self-improvement will see things improve. Besides, tai chi and qigong simply make you feel good. Who doesn't want to feel good? Tai chi is a journey, a healthful journey, a way to a better life and an ageless life.

1

Mind, Body, Brain, Healing

What Matters in Our Lives?

For many years, I have been focused on treating disease. I was trained this way. All doctors, Eastern and Western, are trained to treat disease. I always thought that was what medicine was about. Over the past fifteen years, I have shifted from treating only disease, to treating the whole person. This happened partially because I was not happy with the healthcare system here in the United States, particularly because I was not satisfied with doctors who would spend only five to ten minutes with me and then simply give me a prescription without truly understanding what was going on with my health. I expected that doctors would explain to me why I had this problem, how I would be helped, and what I could do to prevent it from recurring. I then started attending conferences, workshops, lectures, and furthering my reading to understand more about the body. Learning on my own, I started to integrate everything had learned, from Eastern to Western, and to use all this information to help my patients. I found that I grew spiritually, intellectually, and practically in my healing ability as all these viewpoints came together. When my patients were seemingly miraculously improved, I was convinced that my strategy and approaches were right.

For the past five years, I have started to focus on some of my own issues, particularly my brain health, in order to get the most benefit and enjoyment in my own life. I need my brain for living, for conducting business, for creating new methods to achieve health and fitness, for teaching, for healing,

1

for helping others, and for fighting my own aging process. It may sound like I'm doing this all for myself, but actually I am merely the subject of my own experimental research. I am doing all this both to heal myself and to find out if my right-brain dominance can really change. After years of practice in tai chi and qigong, other exercises I've created, as well as other methods I've learned, I now realize that my abilities have changed in many ways: I had fear before, but not anymore; I had anger before, and now it's all gone; I had high expectations for myself, as well as for my family; now I only do the work I love and let others be whoever they want to be. I used to be very stubborn, but now I can let things go much more easily. I used to be skeptical, but now I am open to everything. I tended to fight to try to win if I thought I was right about something, but now I'd rather enjoy the peace; it really doesn't matter who is right and who is not (there is no absolute right and wrong anyway). I used to think I knew everything, but now I know I am still learning every day, and I have so much more to learn. All these experiences and benefits are evidence that our minds, bodies, brains, and the ways we heal are interrelated, and all are important.

Many things can cause stress and cause us to age prematurely. Stress is such a hazard to life, health, healing, and learning; it affects our brains and memories too. Stress can come from work, from home, from physical ailments, from diet, from negative thoughts, from politics, from financial burden, from lack of support, from dealing with unprofessional and irresponsible people, from worrying about retirement, from relationships, from fear, from driving and traffic, from children, parents, and spouse, from the news, from bills and taxes, from the environment, from so many things. This causes tension in our bodies and affects energy flow, which then affects our health from head to toe, including everything from poor productivity to memory loss, depression, heart disease, stroke, and cancer. Other ailments caused by stress include headaches, insomnia, anxiety, back pain, chest pain, hypertension, poor immune system, indigestion, irritable bowel syndrome, substance abuse, anger, social withdrawal, and much more.

No matter how many institutes and facilities focus on stress reduction, the amount of stress is no less than before. People who teach stress reduction are no less stressed than the rest. High technology neither relieves our stress, nor reduces the tension in our bodies, but it can make us lazy in a way. We get too much information, too much stimulation, too much negativity that troubles our minds. Our minds are too busy, It's no wonder many people forget things. We become distracted and don't pay attention to our feelings, our bodies, or our health. We become disconnected and don't know how to protect ourselves or our health. We cannot overcome our emotions; we don't know the right foods to eat or how much food we are supposed to put into our stomach; we don't know how to breathe or how to relax; we become depleted. If something is not right in our bodies, we call a doctor ASAP. If the doctors are too busy with the quantity of patients, the quality in the healthcare they provide is doubtless diminished. Perhaps you have heard this saying: *If you want to stay healthy, stay away from doctors.* This is why.

We are not aware of our own energy. But we do notice other people's energy, others' mistakes, others' failures or successes, others' problems, others' activities, others' lifestyles, and so on. Here is my point, if we don't start paying attention to ourselves, we'll never be able to understand ourselves. We won't be able to solve problems. We won't be able to move forward and we cannot advance ourselves. We cannot heal ourselves if we don't understand ourselves. I remember when I pointed out a mistake someone made in my office, the response was "not me". I would be happy to hear "It wasn't me, but I should pay attention to avoid this in the future". We use a keyboard more often than talking to a live person. We think we don't need to talk to a live person, because our voices can just go through a wire to anyone, anywhere in the world. Many of us are expert at chatting through the computer. When there is a chance of meeting a real person or people, we don't know how to socialize anymore, or we are intimidated to meet people, or we are fearful. Let's face it—we are stuck. Soon we won't know how to calculate any more; we won't need to use our brains much anymore. The bad part is that when dementia hits us, there will be no return.

But there is good news. There has been a great deal of interest in studying the brain as our methods of measurement and our knowledge has increased in recent years. In 1993, journalist Bill Moyers did a program on public television called *Healing and the Mind*. It had a good influence on Americans. Joan Borysenko's *Minding the Body, Mending the Mind* also influenced a large number of Americans. There are many other holistic thinking physicians who have become widely popular, including the doctors Christiane Northrup, Deepak Chopra, Andrew Weil, Wayne W. Dyer, and Dr. Oz. Still, Americans continue to have multiple health problems. Something else needs to be addressed.

There is no doubt that the mind can affect the body and can even heal the body. In my practice, I teach people how to build a strong mind and then use their mind to help with the healing of their body's illness. But interestingly, I have to teach how to use the body to heal the mind as well. In my experience, this technique has proven itself to work much better than the former in some cases. Sometimes the mind cannot heal the body—this can be found in people who are really stuck and cannot change their mindset at all. Sometimes the mind just won't bend or go in the right direction. We have to find another way. And that is to use the body to heal the mind.

The Body Can Heal the Mind

After many years of working with patients, treating patients, teaching patients, and observing patients, I developed my own theory: Body-Brain-Mind-Healing. My idea is to use physical exercises and movement to stimulate the brain and get the brain chemicals activated. By balancing the left and right sides of the brain, upper and lower brain, cross brain, frontal and back brain, through body movements and bringing new information to the brain, we help brain cells communicate with each other. Once the brain is activated and balanced, it guides the mind in the right direction, directing the physical body toward positive behaviors and positive activities. Then the healing begins.

What happens in the complicated human body involves a wholeness that results from many chain reactions. The mind is not the only player. To instigate a chain reaction, something needs to initiate the mind; to get it on the right track, something needs to make the mind work better. The mind can be stuck somewhere in the past, or unable to find a reason for things that happened. Stress can make the mind confused, misled, vulnerable, and debilitated. This is not because our minds are bad or weak, nor because we are stupid. It is because the chemicals in our brains are not balanced; the emotion centers in our brains are not balanced, and so our minds are unbalanced. Fortunately no matter how stuck our minds may be, our bodies can still move. You see everyone walking, getting about, doing things, but you cannot see their underlying health problems. If you can walk and do things, even housework or driving, you can certainly move your body enough to enjoy the variety of exercises proposed here. If you move your body in an energetic way every day, you can change your life and your health.

A patient once asked me, "Why are we here on this planet? What is the purpose of our lives?" If these questions sound a little depressing, try to understand there are things that make us think this way. There were times, when people struggled to survive starvation. Now, some still struggle, not for survival, but to be healthy and to deal effectively with stress. Human beings are born with intelligence, but not with information. Some times too much information can mess up our intelligence. But right information can bring more intelligence. So I told her, "We were born to listen to ourselves: we eat when we are hungry, we sleep when we are tired, we cry when we are uncomfortable, we scream when we are in danger. We lose these basic skills as we grow up, but if we learn to be aware of what is going on with our energy, our body, our mind, our brain, then the next step is to respond, and to restore the balance of our energy, mind, and brain." I almost wanted to reply this way: God made us and God wants us live well.

I have been quite successful in being able to incorporate tai chi, qigong, and other types of body movements into my patient care. Combining and integrating these treatment modalities into a whole package, along with teaching and guiding patients, has brought my healthcare practice to a much higher level. The results: healing, learning, and personal development have changed many Americans' lives. I believe people need this kind integration in our health care system, and it would save a lot of money and make more sense. What really matters in our lives? It's not a big house, not millions dollars in the bank, not the perfect job, not fame. It is your mind, your body, your brain, and your wellbeing. Because when you have these, you have everything. Let's see how much benefit we can get from these ancient Chinese exercises.

Begin Your Journey

In my daily observation of people and after practicing natural healthcare for over twenty-one years, I have noticed one thing that many people cannot overcome, and that is fear. Fear can make you unable to see things in a global or multidimensional way. It prohibits you from moving forward. It prohibits you from seeing the possibilities and discovering your potential. If you open your mind to possibilities, and you are willing to try everything you can, you will find yourself in a different place. From reading books, magazines, and the Internet, you get vast information. But you don't know which information is right. Until you try it yourself, you can't really feel the experience. It may be a bad experience, a good experience, or a so-so experience; maybe it's just a different experience. No matter what experience you have, you learn a lot more than you think.

Healing is the same way; I have had many people tell me that they had a bad experience with their doctor or other medical practitioners. (Though I am sure these medical professionals did the best they can). However, because of their experiences, these people learned how to find answers for themselves, how to take care themselves, and how to search to find their healing paths— what works, what doesn't work. Some people tell me they cannot change the way they live and the way they eat, because this is the way they were brought up. They don't seem to understand that changing is how we develop, how we move forward. Changing expands our knowledge, and allows us to improve. After teaching tai chi and qigong for so many years, I have seen how students changed, including those who said that they could not. This shows that these ancient exercises and physical movements can really change people.

All you need to do is to open your mind to everything, to all that is, and you will open to new possibilities, new opportunities, and a new way of life.

2

Understanding
Tai Chi and Qi Gong

Even though this book is about combating brain aging, I continue talking about Tai Chi and Qi Gong. This is because there are so many benefits for our brain inherent in these exercises.

Tai chi chuan is an ancient Chinese martial arts exercise that has been practiced for centuries. It is known to be a special physical exercise for improving physical health, spiritual health, emotional health, mental health, disease prevention, healing, anti-aging, and self-defense. It is a well-rounded and well-balanced form of exercise. The slow, circular movements require mental concentration and breath control and allow you to move your internal energy, or life force, with your *intention*. The Chinese word for this life force is *qi* (chi). Moving *qi* empowers your body and calms your mind; we call this meditation in motion. It has been proven for centuries that tai chi practice offers great health benefits, including improvement in circulation, metabolism, flexibility, posture, mental concentration, immune function, daily energy level, digestion and absorption, emotional balance, self-awareness, relationships, harmony in your life, and more. From decades of observation and study, it has been shown that tai chi has great benefits to our brains. Tai chi is not just for seniors; it is an exercise for all ages, all races, all religions, all men and women. It is a gift from the Chinese culture, and we can all benefit from it, cherish it, and use it to nourish our energy.

Tai chi helps prevent brain aging. This is why people who practice tai chi over their lifetimes have good overall health. They are multitalented, clear minded, and logical in their thinking and reasoning. They are more creative, have more awareness, and have better skills in dealing with life's challenges.

Qigong (chi gung, Qi Gong, qi gong) is also an ancient Chinese exercise and shares many benefits with tai chi. However, qigong is an easier form of internal energy exercise for health, wellbeing, anti aging, and healing. Qigong is easier to learn and easier to practice than tai chi. The beauty of qigong is that you get results sooner. But both of these exercises are part of anti brain aging practice. For more information about qigong, see my previous book, *Natural Healing with Qigong,* available online and from any bookstore.

What Is Tai Chi?

Tai in Chinese means "bigger than big." *Chi* is not actually the correct word. The correct word should be *Ji. Ji* means extreme. The correct combination for *tai chi* in Chinese is *tai ji chuan. Chuan* is "boxing" or "fist," Altogether, it means grand force boxing, and tai chi certainly has its martial aspect. In the United States, most people just say *tai* chi and skip the *chuan*. It is easier to say, and most of us use it for health anyway, not for fighting.

Tai chi is an *art,* a beautiful art of *motion.* Performing tai chi is like dancing in the clouds. That is why it intrigues people from all over the world. Lovely to watch, it has entertainment value as it is presented internally and externally. This is why you get pleasure from your self as well as from others doing it. I call this kind of pleasure a natural tranquilizer. Unlike other tranquilizers, tai chi is no depressant. Even when things cause people to be depressed, they can quickly use tai chi to activate and redirect the energy, eliminating the depressed mood.

Tai chi is also a form of *meditation,* sometimes called walking meditation or moving meditation. This kind of meditation helps you to focus on the present moment, on your own energy center. You can simply detach yourself from old, disturbing memories. It helps you to relieve stress, untangle your troubled life, and get rid of much of the junk that might be interfering with your happiness.

Tai chi is an *energy workout* that builds your strength both internally and externally. Qigong is also thought of as an energy workout, and tai chi is considered its highest level. These kinds of energy practice can improve energy and blood flow in your body, enhance your immune function, and improve your daily energy level and mental sharpness.

Tai chi is a *training of discipline and focus.* This type of training and discipline can help you to improve many things that happen in your life. It can also help you to reach your future goals once you develop this discipline.

Tai chi is a *martial art,* derived from the whole body of martial arts. In every movement of tai chi, you can find a martial application that can be used for self-defense. As your practice proceeds to higher levels and you continue to study tai chi in-depth, you will notice this more and develop these self-defense skills.

Tai chi is *preventive medicine*—energy medicine or natural healing medicine, because it enhances your self-healing ability, balances your energy, and prevents disease. For people who have chronic ailments where conventional medicine offers no relief, tai chi can assist healing. For people who have cancer, tai chi is an excellent natural medicine that enhances the immune system. Tai chi is also a social medicine. Since it teaches us to focus on ourselves and strengthen our own energy, it prevents violence and other social problems.

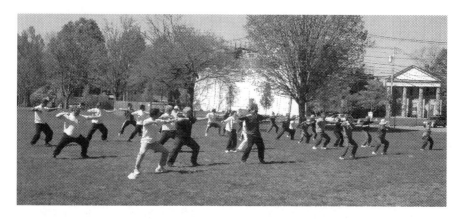

Mind-Body-Spirit

Learning and practicing tai chi and qi gong (Qi Gong) is a wonderful lifestyle. People from all over the world practice tai chi and qi gong for its health benefits to the mind, the body, and the spirit. Tai chi is a mind-body-spirit exercise, whereas most Western style exercises are mainly focused on developing the body.

The *mind* controls the logical part of our existence and determines how we walk straight, read, analyze data, use computers, solve problems, and create and make things happen. The *body* is the physical part of our existence, doing the eating, sleeping, walking, jogging, cooking, and other physiological functions. And the *spirit* is the meaningful part of our existence; this is where our hopes, our dreams, our fears, our love, and our hate are expressed. All of these are equally important. Tai chi has the potential to bridge these separate parts by putting the practitioner in a state of mind where the connections between the three aspects of the whole are made clear. While tai chi exercises the body directly, it has subtle effects on body chemistry in general, and on brain chemistry in particular, thus affecting mood and indirectly affecting the spirit. It requires concentration and attention to detail while being practiced, so we are literally exercising the mind as well.

Tai chi touches all aspects of the whole person at the same time, reinforcing the notion that these so-called separate parts are but different aspects of the same concept. Tai chi helps open the body's energy pathways when practiced through mind, body, and spirit. It is not enough to simply copy the physical movements. You must incorporate them with the other parts of yourself through relaxation, concentration, study of ancient text, meditation, and dedication to your practice.

Jing, Qi, Shen

In Chinese medicine, there are three fundamental substances called *jing, qi, shen*. They in some way refer to our Western terms *body, mind, spirit, and* work side-by-side to keep us healthy.

Jing refers to a fundamental substance in the body, stored in the kidney. *Jing* is usually translated as *essence* and has a very close relationship to the Western term gene, or genetic material. It is crucial to the development of the individual throughout life. It is inherited at birth and allows us to develop from childhood to adulthood and then into old age. It governs growth, reproduction, and development, promotes kidney *qi* and works with *qi* to help protect the body from external pathogens. Any developmental disorder such as learning difficulties and physical disabilities in children may be due to a deficiency of *jing* from birth. Other disorders such as infertility, poor memory, a tendency to get sick or catch colds, and allergies may also be due to deficiency of *jing*.

Qi refers to vital energy or life-force flow in the body, like the electric flow in a wire. There are various types of *qi* in the body working together to keep our physical atmosphere in harmony. *Qi* has a very close relationship to human metabolism, immune function, digestion, absorption, emotion, breathing, mental clarity, and more. Qi is present internally and externally and controls the function of all parts of the body. *Qi* is the motor of the body, just like the motor in the car. *Qi* keeps us moving and functioning, keeps us warm, and protects us against sickness. Everything we do involves *qi*. Walking, eating, laughing, crying, playing sports, working, hiking, and writing are all related to *qi*. *Qi* affects our life every day. We cannot see the *qi* in the body, but we can feel it. We can feel when our energy is low and when it is high. We can sense if we are optimistic or depressed; we can feel if our bodies are out of balance. *Qi* is very important in the body and in life.

Shen refers to our spiritual energy, our highest consciousness, a reconnection with universal energies.

The English word *spirit* has many differing meanings and connotations, but commonly refers to a supernatural being or essence, transcendent and therefore metaphysical in its nature. *The Concise Oxford Dictionary* defines it as "the non-physical part of a person." For many people, however, spirit, like *soul*, forms a natural part of a being, not a transcendence of some sort. Such people may identify spirit with *mind* or with *consciousness* or with the *brain*.

Christian theology uses the term *Shen* or *Spirit* (capitalized) to describe God, or aspects of God—as in the *Holy Spirit*, referring to a *Triune God* (Trinity). In popular theological terms, the individual human spirit (singular, lowercase) is a deeply situated aspect of the soul, subject to spiritual growth and change, the very seat of emotion and desire, and the transmitting organ by which humans can contact God. In a rare theological definition, it consists of higher consciousness enclosing the soul. Christian Scientists use "Spirit" as one of the seven synonyms for God, as in "Principle, Mind, Soul, Spirit, Life, Truth, and Love."

Some people refer to *shen* as a Soul. In Chinese medicine theory, *shen* and soul are two different things with some similarities. Soul is the immaterial or *eternal* part of a living being, commonly held to be *separable in existence* from the body. Shen in traditional Chinese medicine (TCM) is the *lifted* or *energized eternal* part of a living being.

Jing, qi, and *shen* are built upon one another. Proficient *jing* leads to balanced *qi*. Balanced *qi* creates better *shen*. Improving the circulation of *qi* enhances and strengthens *Jing*, as well as lifting *shen*. Good *shen* can control and connect to *qi*, and be a guide to create more balanced *qi*. The cycle goes on and on, affecting each other in both positive and negative ways.

By practicing tai chi and qi gong, you strengthen the storage of *jing*, smooth the flow of the *qi*, and build better *shen*. You improve physical health, psychological well being, and expand and enhance the spirit.

During my many years of teaching, I have seen our students succeed in decreasing their stress level and increasing their overall health. They have increase in flexibility, stamina, balance, poise, and skill in interpersonal interactions, and mental focus. More information can be found below.

The Benefits of Tai Chi in Four Major Parts

— Physical

You have enhanced stamina and strength, a balanced immune system, a harmonized organ system, and you are preventing disease. From teaching tai chi over twenty years, I have seen many students improve in their physical condition; they are sick less frequently even in flu season, are physically stronger, and their chronic issues have improved. Many times, students have told me, "Everyone in my family gets sick, except me," or they say, "I haven't been sick for several years." It is especially satisfying when I hear these things from senior citizens. It is easy to see that their overall health has improved, and some have even reduced their medications. There are more and more studies on the benefits of tai chi appearing nationally and internationally.

In the United States, scientists studied tai chi's effect on improving balance and preventing falls in the elderly; this is just a side benefit of tai chi. No doubt there will be more in-depth studies in the future on many of the important health benefits of tai chi, such as preventing heart disease, reducing blood pressure, relieving depression and anxiety, and others.

— Mental

Practicing or learning Tai Chi definitely will make you calm and less stressed. In my book *Tai Chi for Depression,* I explain clearly how this works. People who practice Tai Chi for a lifetime don't have mental issues. Or if something happens dramatically, they can deal with it with the right attitude.

The anti-aging benefits of tai chi practice give you mental clarity, so your reasoning improves and you are able to do things in an efficient way. Your creativity is awakened and can make your life more multicolored and livelier. Your renewed alertness helps you to keep relationships and friendships strong. As we have all experienced, it can be frustrating to talk to someone who cannot understand what you are saying, even when you have tried to explain it a dozen times. We get frustrated when telling someone something many times, and they still cannot remember. It is even more frustrating when we want and try to help, but feel helpless. Poor memory may not only affect you, it can affect the people who live with you, deal with you, and work with you on a daily basis. For instance, someone may ask you to do something and you agree to do it, but then it doesn't get done because you forgot. This might not bother you, but the person who asked you to perform the task is waiting for this and maybe it is important to them. Of course this person will be frustrated but can not say much about it. I had a friend complain about his girlfriend. He gave a gift to her but she denied she received it. He could not believe this, but had to admit she must have forgotten. This is my reason for doing tai chi, teaching tai chi; to keep my own brain healthy. And it works; my memory is *better* than it was when I was younger.

— Emotional

People who seriously practice tai chi tend to have more stable emotions. They display an evenness of mood, remaining more calm and peaceful. They are able to better control their emotions during conflict and stressful situations. They are able to let things go more easily. This is because of smooth energy flow in their organ system, as well as the brain benefits from tai chi and qigong practice. There will be more details on this in chapter two's "How Tai Chi and Qi Gong Prevent Brain Aging and Memory Loss".

— Spiritual

The spirit is that which is beyond the ordinary; it is an intangible, higher consciousness that never dies. It connects us with ourselves, both physically and emotionally. Spirit defines who we are, how we think, *what* we think, and how we interrelate with the universe. It also describes both how we view God and our relationship with God. Spirit is a special energy that cannot be seen, heard, touched, or otherwise experienced *materially*. It can however be felt or experienced *internally* by ourselves, by people around us, and even by animals. I have a dog, a lovely dog. When my spirit energy is poor, she can sense it. She comes to sit near me and tries to be very quiet. When my spirit energy is high, she wants to play. Fortunately, my spirit energy is pretty good most of the time. Our spirits are on a constant path towards enlightenment, constantly weighing, experiencing, and reacting to life's yin (receptive, dark, feminine) and yang (active, bright, masculine) sides.[1]

The meditative aspect of tai chi allows us to tap into and activate our spirits. Our minds translate what our bodies feel as we move, and interpreting our spirits at the same time. Our minds integrate what we sense about the world in order to move our body accordingly. Tai chi is also an expression of spirit by way of the mind and body. When we practice as a group, our spirits coalesce. Our spirits accumulate the group energy, which we then express in unity, or *as one*. Whether we practice tai chi alone or with others, we are connecting body, mind, and spirit with the whole universe.

Tai chi is known as a meditative art form. And like meditation, practicing tai chi helps to balance the spirit, as well as balancing our own yin and yang

---

1   Please refer to my book *Simple Chinese Medicine* for information about yin and yang.

aspects. It allows us not to be absorbed or overtaken by *negative* spirit, or negative energy. It is as though tai chi helps us to create a shield against negative energy. We tend to gravitate more toward people with positive spirit, and we more easily embrace it (positive spirit).

Mind, body, and spirit connect with each other in an important way. When you let your mind, body, and spirit work together, you appear at peace with yourself. You become aware of your energy and feel the effects of tai chi in your body. Additionally, you enjoy the sensation of satisfaction that comes from performing the movements. You become more and more familiar with many other positive aspects as your practice proceeds. This is not an easy journey, but it is very rewarding, especially as the benefits are manifest in later life.

Tai chi has already changed my life in numerous ways. It is as much of an energy medicine for me, as it is for other people. It is also an energy medicine *science,* which Western scientists are finally starting to recognize. The best way of learning this true art of healing and wellbeing is by experience. To find out how much you can get from tai chi practice, start your journey today. I know it will be wonderful.

Daoist Practice:

Tai chi, qi gong, and Chinese medicine all come from Daoist (also Taoist) principles. In Daoist philosophy, everything on the earth has two opposite sides: yin and yang.[2] In order to keep the balance of the cosmos, it is important to keep the balance of the yin and the yang. In times of tragedy, chaos, and instability, as well as in cases of health problems, we will often see an imbalance of yin and yang. When practicing tai chi, you are actually *walking the Daoist path.* Daoism helps you to be more relaxed, let go easier, keep an inner peace. There are many versions of the Dao (Tao) and Daoist translations in bookstores. I recommend that you find a copy and read a chapter a day for "bedtime learning."

Higher Level Qi Gong

As a type of *qi* practice, tai chi is a higher-level qi gong, an internal energy workout. Both require full concentration, breath control, and specific positions and movements of the body, but tai chi's movements are much more intricate. Much more discipline is involved. To know the difference between tai chi

---

2   You can find much information on yin and yang in my book *Simple Chinese Medicine.*

and qigong, please see my book *Natural Healing with Qigong* as further reference.

Tai Chi—The Perfect Exercise?

The following article by [Bill Douglas[3], the founder of World Tai Chi and Qi Gong Day,] provides an interesting discussion on the growing popularity of tai chi attributable to a growing body of research demonstrating its benefits:

> *Tai Chi & Qigong have exploded across the media landscape recently. Time Magazine in an article on Tai Chi benefits called Tai Chi "the perfect exercise." While The Wall Street Journal recently did a front page lifestyle story entitled Qigong The Next Yoga: A Sweat Free Workout— Tiger Woods' Secret Weapon?*
>
> *So, why all the buzz on Tai Chi & Qigong? Partly because today's high stressed fast moving population is seeking, not only health & fitness, but serenity. Serenity may sound superficial in today's busy world, but that aspect of Tai Chi, may be why it is increasingly utilized in healthcare, corporate wellness, education, and even in prison and drug rehabilitation programs.*
>
> *The current hubbub about Tai Chi & Qigong may be that we are only now seeing the breaking of a tsunami wave of growing evidence unearthed by western medical research that has been quietly building for the last decade. Qigong is a Traditional Chinese medical/health practice that directly translated means "breathing exercise," or "energy exercise." Tai Chi is a sophisticated form of moving qigong, which involves a series of choreographed movements done in a relaxed and flowing way. Both have gained increasing attention by western medical researchers in the last decade that has been gaining steam, and resulted in more research dollars going toward discovering their benefits. The National Institute of Mental Health has increased funding to further research these ancient, yet modern, health techniques.*
>
> *A couple of such study's findings, one a ten year study through Harvard, Yale, and Emory Universities, stunned researchers when they*

3   Bill Douglas is the Founder of World Tai Chi & Qigong Day www.WorldTaiChiDay.org (celebrated annually in nearly 70 nations), and the Tai Chi Expert at www.DrWeil.com. Bill was the 2009 Inductee into the Internal Arts Hall of Fame and his best selling Tai Chi book, *The Complete Idiot's Guide to T'ai Chi & Qigong*, and DVD program, *Anthology of T'ai Chi & Qigong*, are internationally acclaimed.

discovered that the gentle, slow, relaxing, low impact Tai Chi improved the balance of practitioners profoundly, reducing their risk of falling by 47.5%. Another found that Tai Chi offered significant cardiovascular benefits, roughly the same benefits as moderate impact aerobics. Yet, another study sited in the Hawaii Medical Journal asserted that Tai Chi increased breathing capacity and relieved back and neck aches in practitioners.

The pain relief and low impact aspects of Tai Chi was good news for everyone, but offered even more hope for those suffering from rheumatoid arthritis (RA). Tai Chi being a weight bearing exercise offered the potential advantages of stimulating bone growth and strengthening connective tissue. The only concern was if those with rheumatoid arthritis could handle a weight bearing exercise without exacerbation of joint symptoms, but the American Journal of Physical Medicine and Rehabilitation reported on a study that found people with RA who practiced a specially tailored form of Tai Chi suffered "no" significant exacerbation of joint symptoms. This was great news, not just for RA sufferers but for all maturing baby boomers looking for a health regimen that is kind to the joints.

Surprisingly, given its gentle nature, Tai Chi burns a significant amount of calories as well, 280 per hour. To understand how significant this is, realize that down-hill skiing burns about 350 per hour. Yet, Tai Chi is gentle enough to be done in business clothes in the office without even breaking a sweat. Which is one reason Tai Chi and Qigong are increasingly being used in corporate wellness programs. However, there are perhaps even more important reasons Tai Chi is being used, not only in corporate wellness, but health care, education, and even prisons and drug rehabilitation institutions.

Tai Chi provides a grouping of benefits that helps reduce productivity losses in employees; may reduce health care costs preemptively; enables students to focus; and also helps to empower those rehabilitating from drug abuse, etc;. to evolve more healthy productive lifestyles. This is the result of mood homeostasis Tai Chi practice fosters. The Journal of Psychosomatic Research reports a Tai Chi study's findings, "[Test Subjects] reported less tension, depression, anger, fatigue, confusion and state-anxiety; they felt more vigorous, and in general they had less total mood disturbance."

Given that 70 to 85% of illness sending patients to the doctor are rooted in unmanaged stress, and that US business is estimated to be losing upwards of $300 billion annually due to unmanaged stress, Tai Chi's potential mood-stabilizing benefits are gaining increasing attention. In *education the rise in ADD and ADHD symptoms in our nation's youth has peaked interest in Tai Chi by some education professionals. This may be partly due to a recent study from the University of Miami School of Medicine finding that Tai Chi provided substantial symptom reduction in students suffering from Attention Deficit and Hyperactivity Disorder (ADHD).*

In light of the multi-dimensional benefits these ancient health practices offer, which are now being validated by modern health research, the Time Magazine description of Tai Chi as "the perfect exercise" may be very accurate for this ancient mind/body health technique.

From the above article, we see that Western science is more and more looking at natural body/energy exercise for its benefits. Many studies show the physical benefits of tai chi. I know soon they will be looking into its benefits for the human brain—to find out why tai chi practitioners stay sharp and alert even in old age.

Tai chi is a lifestyle, a special exercise involving sophisticated movements. Some people might become frustrated, because short-term use does not provide long-lasting benefits. Brief participation can give you only a little taste of tai chi. Learning tai chi also requires having a good instructor who can teach you all the aspects of tai chi, the true nature of tai chi, and not just the movements. This supplemental knowledge includes the history, principles, and foundation of practice, *qi* practice, inner focus practice, breathing practice, and more. This way, you can truly get the maximum benefits you desire.

Not Just for Senior Citizens—Tai Chi Is for Everyone

A common misconception that I hear is that "tai chi is for old people." Well sure, many seniors are limited in what exercises they can do, and tai chi is slow and gentle and has a very low risk of injury; therefore, it is ideally suited for seniors. But in truth, tai chi is good for everyone, including children.

Learning tai chi is actually a little easier for younger people, who can perform the more extreme movements, such as maximum stretching for the long lunges, bending knees for the low stances. Older people will want to find an instructor with a great deal of experience teaching seniors who knows how to modify the positions for their abilities. Seniors do not need to bend knees as much, for example; instead, they can just unlock the knee.

The main thing is that everyone who continues to practice tai chi throughout their lives will see tangible results. You will notice that life seems easier and your outlook is much more positive. All of your achievements will be greater from having a well-balanced mind and body.

Many young people like to practice tai chi to focus on the martial aspect, so they can enhance their fighting abilities and power. The world famous martial art practitioner Jet Lee won five gold medals at China Martial Art competitions many years ago. He studied tai chi from China's highly respected teacher Feng Zhi Qiang, who was also my mentor. There is true value in tai chi as a martial art. I enjoy watching Jet Lee's martial arts performances in his movies. His fighting skills are remarkable.

Older people prefer to use tai chi for fitness and longevity, to prevent an existing illness from getting worse, and to prevent illness from occurring. Still, you might see some older tai chi practitioners who are also practicing the martial aspects of this art.

Some people (both Chinese and American) complain that tai chi seems too slow, and it doesn't look like much physical exercise, or it doesn't have the feeling of a workout. There may be numerous reasons why they think this way. This may be because the instructor did not give complete instructions, or the instructor did not give enough warm up exercises; maybe the students are not practicing long enough, or maybe the students did not follow instructions well. Practicing tai chi is very physical; you may be surprised at how much of a workout you can actually get from tai chi practice and how much physical power you can generate from tai chi practice. Tai chi's workout is invisible, subtle. It is slow for a reason—slow-motion, concentration—but it has a power that is very strong and rooted. Patience and persistence are the keys to success in tai chi.

In our modern, fast-paced society, we need a slow and balanced exercise to help regulate our lives. If we are busy all the time and have no breaks or rest, our bodies will be over-driven, and just like an over-driven car, it will break down sooner than it has to. When body chemicals like adrenalin and noradrenalin are at a high level for a long time, the heart is over-stimulated. In such a state, we are prone to heart disease, high blood pressure, and rapid aging. If we work our minds too hard, think too hard, or think every minute, it slows down our creativity, productivity and causes brain aging. With non-stop life styles or high stress life styles, we will also have many other problems, including cholesterol problems, energy problems, low immune function, cancer, and many other illnesses. A dog runs fast, and its life span is less than eighteen years. The turtle moves slow, and its life span is around 100 to 150 years, depending on its species. Perhaps there's something to that. The human lifespan can vary—how long do you want yours to be? The most important thing is not just to live longer, but to live better. If I have a poor quality life, I don't need to live longer; but if I have a quality life, yes, I want to enjoy my life and live longer. By eating well, focusing on preventive work and practicing tai chi and qigong, you can prolong your life and always improve it.

Because tai chi promotes internal strength by building strong *qi*, it can be a powerful training tool for martial artists. Many martial art schools offer tai chi classes for both martial arts people and non-martial arts people. You don't have to be a martial artist to benefit from tai chi. People of all ages and abilities practice this all-round well-being exercise, including people with disabilities and ailments, who use it as therapy.

How Tai Chi and Qigong Assist Human Healing

In the Chinese healing system, your mind and your body cannot be separated. Your body can affect your mind, and your mind can affect your body. Your energy pathways that go through your body also go through your brain and affect all parts of the brain including the neurochemicals.

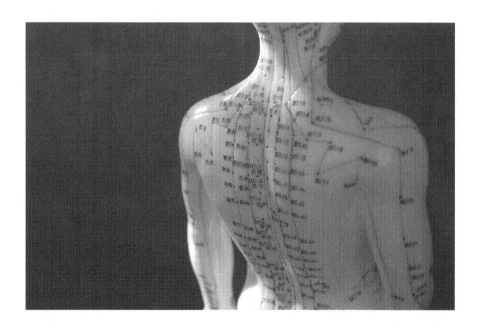

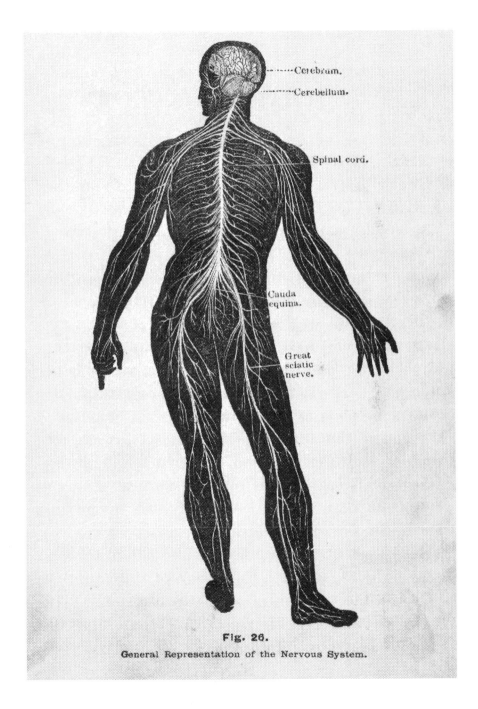

Fig. 26.

General Representation of the Nervous System.

Both tai chi and qi gong work on internal energy. Internal energy brings harmony to the organ system. The harmonious organ system helps to balance biochemistry, hormones, and metabolism in the body. This is how your healing ability is enhanced. When you have surgery, your wound may be healed in days or weeks, even months. It all depends on your level of healing ability. When you catch a cold, you may recover in days, weeks, or months; this also depends on our healing ability. If your healing ability is strong, you can heal any illness. (I know some people don't believe this, especially medical people—I was one of them.) If your healing ability is poor or weak, your chance of healing is poor. It might take longer to heal, or you could even lose your life. Using tai chi and qi gong to improve your healing ability provides a powerful reason to start your tai chi journey. Here is how tai chi and qi gong are associated with healing:

— Cardiovascular Support

The slow and meditative movements of tai chi and qi gong help to smooth the flow of the energy. Tai chi and qi gong elevates the function of the vagus nerve system, which has a big effect on reducing stress and preventing heart disease and hypertension. We discussed previously, *qi* is the motor of the body. Just like a car, a bigger car with a bigger motor will go faster and have more power; a smaller car will go slower and have less power. If *qi* in the body is strong and balanced, your body and circulation system will be strong and you will be less likely to develop circulatory and vascular diseases. For many years in China, the rates of heart disease and hypertension have been low. One of the reasons for this is that people pay attention to and work on improving their bodies' *qi* circulation. They also maintain a healthy diet, have a balanced and active social life, and often walk from place to place, instead of driving. Recently, the situation has changed: there is now more heart disease, hypertension, diabetes, obesity, and other problems. There are also more cars. This does not mean we don't need cars.

— Respiratory Support

One of the most important benefits, which is also easy for Westerners to understand, is the increased oxygen level in the blood and organ system. Both tai chi and qi gong require deep breathing. With each slow and deep breath, you bring more oxygen to your body, to your lungs, and to your bloodstream. Your blood travels to all parts of the body, your brain, heart, kidneys, liver, stomach, intestines, spleen, reproductive system, muscle system, glands, etc. The more oxygen you bring into the body, the better the quality of the body's health.

Tai chi and qi gong not only increases the oxygen flow in the body but also increases its usage by organs and tissue. That is why tai chi and qi gong is considered a natural anti-oxidant. This also contributes to delaying the aging process. By practicing deep breathing, your lung energy improves. To use a Western explanation, it is known that when lung capacity increases, we get more air, and so more oxygen. On one trip to China, I had my friends examine my chest x-ray film. One friend practices internal medicine and the other is a radiologist. Both of them told me it was amazing that even though I had chronic inflammation in my lungs, the amount of air I could breathe was remarkably good. I was disappointed about my inflammation—I was born with poor lung and kidney energy—but I was happy about my lung *function*. This helps bring a good amount of oxygen to my body. I am proof that people who have chronic lung issues can be helped with qi gong and tai chi practice.

These exercises also help to prevent respiratory infection, cold, flu, or any kind of lung disease. In our lungs, there are special antibodies called IgA (immunoglobulin). IgA protects us from respiratory infection. Theoretically, qi gong practice increases the IgA in both quantity and quality. In Chinese medical theory, qi gong practice improves your defensive energy, which is also called protective energy. People who practice qi gong are unlikely to get respiratory diseases and colds. I often feel blessed that I haven't been sick for many years.

— Gastrointestinal Support

Tai chi and qigong improve the autonomic nervous system, including both the sympathetic nervous system and the parasympathetic nervous system. In a later chapter we will find out how important these nervous systems are to our health. The parasympathetic nerves are responsible for internal organs, especially the digestive system. With improved blood circulation, more oxygen gets to the organs; with improved parasympathetic nerve function, your digestive enzymes, the mobility of the digestive track and other digestive chemicals are more likely to stay at healthy levels. When intestine mobility is normal, you have natural cleansing and detoxification.

You know you don't feel well if you cannot go to the bathroom for several days. Maintaining good digestive energy leads to better digestion and absorption. With these advantages, the food you eat will be properly used and transformed to energy; otherwise, the food you eat will not be transformed to energy and you will feel tired even though you may have eaten well. The movements in tai chi and qi gong involves the whole body, you sometimes are doing a gentle massage to your internal organs during practice. This gentle stimulation helps to restore the balance of the digestive organs and prevent digestive disorder.

I have been surprised to find out that there are so many cases of digestive illness in the United States. I have many patients with digestive illnesses, but very few are willing to do tai chi and qi gong. But my patients who have taken my advice and practiced tai chi and qi gong, did improve.

Many people take various supplements trying to help themselves. The supplements can help you if your digestive system can absorb and use the supplements. If you have imbalance in the digestive system, using supplements is rather wasteful, because your supplements are not absorbed or used well either. True masters of tai chi and qi gong rarely have digestive problems. Diligent practice of tai chi can help you to reach your goal of optimal health.

— **Musculoskeletal Support**

Tai chi and qi gong involve the whole body with flexion, contraction, stretching, and multi dimensional movements. Your muscles get a well-rounded exercise. This is especially true with "Therapeutic Qi Gong" (offered in our school in weekly classes as well as in the Qi Gong Instructor Training Program). Your muscles and joints are in constant motion and receive plenty of oxygen from the workout. This not only keeps you fit, but also keeps your muscles and joints healthy. You will have less muscle tension and stiffness. This helps delay muscles and joints from aging and degeneration, and maintains good muscle resiliency and flexibility. Healthy muscles and tendons can also prevent arthritis, fibromyalgia, and tendonitis. Not only will you have fewer aches and pains and less stiffness, but you will also have less chance of a fracture when you fall, because strong and flexible muscles support your bones. Consequently, your body feels younger, and so does your mind.

In 1991, I went to China. As usual, I went to a public park in the early morning, and I saw an eighty-two-year-old woman doing Chinese exercise. In practicing her qi gong, she kicked her leg even higher than I could kick. I then found out she came to this park to do exercise everyday, rain or shine.

I know it is easier to practice in China, because there are so many people doing it in public parks. This, in itself, creates an energy field; you spontaneously do it without hesitation. It is harder in America, not only because it is such a new thing here, but also because people feel self-conscious being in a public place doing exercise. I think that is why we don't see many people doing these exercises outdoors.

— Increase Stamina, Daily Energy Level, and Immune Function:

Tai Chi strengthens the immune system. People who practice tai chi not only improve their balance and coordination, they also improve their immunity. A study[4] at the Neuropsychiatric Institute at the University of California, Los Angeles, showed very interesting results in group of older men and women who took tai chi for forty-five minutes, three days a week. They showed an increase of up to 50 percent of memory T-cells. These are the immune system cells that identify and fight the varicella herpes virus. This is the virus that causes shingles. People who have had chicken pox are vulnerable to shingles because the virus can remain dormant in nerve cells indefinitely. As we get older our immune system get weaker, so the virus can wake up. Then you may have the symptoms shingles, which causes blisters on the skin and is very painful. Results of the study were published in the September 2003 issue of Psychosomatic Medicine.

With improved energy flow, your body is in an optimum state. Your endurance is good and stamina is strong. You will be able to work longer hours and still have good productivity. Because of the balanced chemicals in the body, the immune system tends to be balanced too. People who practice tai chi and qigong have much less chance of getting sick. In my teaching, I have seen many of my students improve their energy levels and immune systems. They rarely catch colds. Even when they have caught colds, they recovered from it more quickly than others.

— Affects on the Nervous System:

As mentioned above, the movements from tai chi and qi gong affect the nervous system, including the central nervous system, peripheral nervous system, and autonomic nervous system. The whole-body exercise incorporates breathing and mental focus, which allows *qi* and blood to flow better to all parts of the body, including the brain. By balancing the biochemicals and neurochemicals in the body and brain, you can be more focused, respond more quickly to learning, think more logically, maintain mental sharpness

---

4   Irwin, Michael R., Pike, Jennifer L., Cole, Jason C., Oxman, Michael N. **Effects of a Behavioral Intervention, Tai Chi Chih, on Varicella-Zoster Virus Specific Immunity and Health Functioning in Older Adults** Psychosom Med 2003 65: 824-830

and alertness, and improve your ability to perform daily tasks with greater ease.

Tai chi and qi gong not only regulate the somatic nervous system, as evidenced by the improved mobility of the muscles and joints, but also improve the autonomic nervous system, including sympathetic and parasympathetic nerve system response. The autonomic nervous system is divided into two opposite functions, and is comprised of the sympathetic and parasympathetic nervous systems. These neural networks control the internal organ systems, glands, blood vessels, and sensory systems. For many years, my focus has been on nervous system and autonomic healing. The healing work I do and the special exercises I create are designed to improve and balance the entire nervous system.

Each deep inhalation stimulates sympathetic activity, whereas each exhalation stimulates parasympathetic activity. The more regulated breathing you practice, the better-balanced autonomic nerve system you will have. That is why qi gong masters have much fewer physical complaints in their lives. They have a very good digestive function as well as a good immune function. This helps explains how tai chi and qi gong have a self-regulating effect on the human body.

There will be more details about the autonomic nervous system in a coming chapter, but suffice it to say that these benefits remain even as you age, which has given me the encouragement to write this book. I have seen many of my friends with declining memories, even some who were very smart at a younger age. On the other hand, I have noticed that my tai chi and qi gong students have less depression and anxiety, less stress, and less confusion in making decisions. It greatly benefits people who have ADD too. I believe if we start to teach children tai chi or qi gong at early ages, it could help them to focus, and they will do better in their academic studies and other activities. They will have healthier mental processes too. Unfortunately, our culture has not paid much attention to support this.

— Correction of Chemical Imbalances

Deep, slow, and regulated breathing helps to harmonize the body's chemistry, including adrenaline, noradrenalin, serotonin, and many other neurochemicals. Many illnesses are caused by chemical or hormonal imbalances. If you use external chemicals to balance the internal chemicals, such as taking a pill to supplement a chemical that is low in the blood, you may actually cause more imbalances by interfering with the body's natural biofeedback response. Our bodies are auto-regulating systems, which allow us to be in balance most of the time. If a certain chemical is low, the auto-regulating system will stimulate the corresponding organ to release more of this particular chemical to balance the level. External chemicals (or pills) suppress this self-regulating response and provide false information to the body, so it stops releasing the very chemical it needs. That is why a person who takes a thyroid hormone pill will usually have to take it for life. If a person uses a pill to supplement the thyroid hormone, the destruction of the self-regulating system of the thyroid gland, pituitary gland, and hypothalamus will result; then his or her thyroid will no longer function. If the person starts to practice tai chi or qi gong consistently or gets acupuncture or Chinese herb treatments, this person has a chance of restoring the self-regulating system. Eventually, the level of the hormones will be normal.

With tai chi and qigong practice, there is definitely a feeling of chemical balance. There is stillness in motion, and there is motion in stillness. If it involved just stillness without any motion, it might be difficult for some people to follow. If it were just motion without stillness, such as a heavy workout offers, we would lose the sense of peace and harmony. Try to practice tai chi and qi gong when you are stressed to see how you feel afterward.

— Other Benefits:

- Both tai chi and qi gong improve metabolism. You rarely see an overweight qigong master or long-time practitioner.

- Improved balance and coordination, which research has shown, helps to prevent falls and injuries.

- People experience improvement in lifestyle and happiness. This is from becoming well-balanced and open-minded. The masters of tai chi and qi gong don't get stressed, because they know how to avoid negative energy.

- Improved learning ability in all fields. We will have more details on this in later chapters.

- Harmony in the working of the organs. This is very important in any field, as well as in health and healing. Please reference my book, *Simple Chinese Medicine*, for information regarding organ teamwork.

- Cancer healing. One very important aspect of tai chi and qi gong practice is its ability to assist cancer healing. It helps to prevent the onset of cancer and prevent cancer relapse. It can also help to heal cancer. I know very few people believe this statement. A majority of people might say, "Yeah, right Doc, this is a joke;

cancer needs chemotherapy, radiation therapy, hormone therapy, steroids therapy, surgery, and more drugs." Sound familiar? But think for a moment: how many cancer patients died, even though they had received these conventional therapies? Common sense shows that your balanced mind is a guide to your balanced body, and your balanced body helps you to heal. Anything can change: your health, your illness, your life too. I could be crippled by my chronic lung inflammation by now, but I am not.

Tai chi and qi gong strengthen the immune system, and a strong immune system helps to fight cancer. People who have a strong immune system die from old age, even if they have cancer cells in their bodies. Only if you have a weak immune system, can the cancer cells grow faster and be more invasive. A weakened immune system caused by some conventional treatments can cause severe infection, which is a main cause of death for cancer patients. Tai chi and qi gong can put patients into a positive state of mind and promote positive thoughts, giving crucial hope for healing. It is like mental training and teaching. Scientists know the mind has immense power with regard to human disease and healing. I have seen this first hand. You may be surprised to know that even I did not believe these things before. Research has now shown that mental training has the power to change the physical structure of the brain.

"...... Mental practice resulted in a similar reorganization" of the brain, Pascual-Leone later wrote. If his results hold for other forms of movement (and there is no reason to think they don't), then mentally practicing a golf swing or a forward pass or a swimming turn could lead to mastery with less physical practice. Even more profound, the discovery showed that mental training had the power to change the physical structure of the brain. (The Brain: How The Brain Rewires Itself TIME: Fri January 19, 2007

(Read more: http://www.time.com/time/magazine/ article/0,9171,1580438,00.html#ixzz0ytKCxti])

In China, people who have cancer always seek treatment from both medicines: conventional and holistic. Most of them do qi gong regularly in addition to using herbal medicine. I have several cancer patients who visit me regularly, and they are doing very well. I highly recommend that if you have cancer, start to use qi gong or tai chi as a life time companion. You will not regret it.

Please keep in mind, tai chi and qi gong are not magic, even though they can provide amazing benefits. All the benefits come from diligent practice, faith, a positive attitude, and patience.

Tai Chi, the True Art of Healing and Wellbeing

As mentioned earlier, when I was starting out as a doctor, my focus was mainly on treating disease. Now, my focus is on teaching people how to prevent disease. This may not seem that impressive, because no one appreciates good health when everything seems fine. But it has incredible value—anyone will appreciate good health when they see others suffering from various illnesses. I have always believed that a preventive approach should be the job of a good doctor. I believe this is what gives a doctor the most value in healthcare. I have come by this wisdom about good health from my lifetime of practice and from teaching and training people in tai chi and qi gong. This is how I can share my experience with people and hopefully more and more people will enjoy the benefits that can be found here.

3

Tai Chi and Brain Fitness

Did you see my watch?
Did you see my wallet?
What time is my appointment?
Where did I put my papers?
I cannot find my keys.
I cannot find my checkbook.
I forgot to go to my class.
I forgot all about my appointment today.
What were you saying?
I cannot find my red shirt.
Where is my cell phone?

Aren't we all familiar with this kind of talk? I have heard these too often. Maybe this is why I am writing this book. Our brains start aging at around age twenty-four. We lose 100,000 brain cells each day, which sounds scary. When we have difficulty with perception and memory, we get frustrated, anxious, even depressed. When we forget something important, it costs us money, time, and energy. In some cases, it can be very disturbing.

Many years ago, a friend of mine was going on a trip. He needed to fly to Germany for work. When he went to check in at the airport, he realized that he had forgotten to bring his airplane ticket and his photo ID. He had to drive forty miles back home to pick them up, because at the time there was no electronic ticketing. Of course, he missed the plane and then had to take a later one. What if there was only one plane that day? Another friend of mine forgot to turn off the stove one day. She accidentally started an oil fire and burned a kitchen cabinet. I have heard stories from my family and friends about their experience of having left their umbrellas behind in stores; left watches, wallets, or jewelry on hotel bedside tables, or couldn't find their tickets for a show. Some people even left credit cards in restaurants. There are so many cases of forgetfulness, some that I have to deal with on a daily basis.

I am not saying that I am perfect; but I am aware that when things need to be worked on. I have seen the difference this kind of thinking has made in my own life. Many people feel that their memory is getting worse, but I am happy to say my memory is just fine, or stayed same as twenty years ago. However, I am sure that I have lost many brain cells.

The sad part is that cases of forgetfulness are appearing in younger and younger people, even teenagers. Maybe it is from our busy lifestyle; maybe it is due to too much on our plates; maybe we are not pointing our brains in the right direction; maybe we are too conservative and unwilling to change; maybe we just cannot focus; maybe kids or younger people use too many electronics that cause them to not use their brain; or maybe we were just born this way.

Everything has two sides; we tend to be more forgetful when we get older, but we also gain some benefits. We are wiser, more mature, more experienced, and have a better understanding of life and career. We also have better social skills. We become willing to learn to improve and to overcome our weaknesses; this is why some people are able to maintain a good memory, while others are not. I have always believed that anything is possible. We should always keep in mind: anything can change, and anything can improve.

I used to be very forgetful in my younger days—due to that genetic issue of weak kidney *qi*. I remember how much I struggled due to my poor health when I was studying in medical school. I struggled to memorize the medical stuff and trying to comprehend. In early years, I sometimes would go back and forth to check if I'd locked my door; sometimes I had to drive back to the office. Several times, I got back to the office and found that the door was unlocked. I did not know if I was the one who forgot, or if it was the other people working with me who forgot. Since there was no evidence, there was no answer. I might have forgotten once, but not *so many* times. At any rate, it gave me the desire to do more work on improving my brain and my memory. I will share with you how I did that with tai chi and qi gong. But first, let's begin with a basic understanding of our brains.

Understanding Our Brains and Brain Aging

The brain is a very special organ with a very complicated wiring system similar to a computer network. This three-pound lump of wrinkled tissue with no observable moving parts directs all parts of the body, including all movement, sensation, thought processing, creativity, emotion, talking, eating, walking, self regulating, breathing, and much more. Our brains are complex and mysterious and present a multitude of challenges to our understanding of its workings. It is so advanced and interesting that it makes us want to explore more. The chemistry in the brain is also very complex. It enables hundreds of different personalities and various emotions to be expressed.

Thousands of scientists have studied the human brain, and they are finding out new things about it every day. Some new findings have replaced old findings, making all our old beliefs questionable. The medical and pharmaceutical industries also study the brain to help them create new drugs to change our brain chemistry and treat mental illness and brain degeneration. Educators study the brain in hope of finding ways to improve learning skills in children and younger adults. I study the brain mainly to improve my own memory and enjoyment of life. Although we may never completely unravel the mystery of the brain, we have found a great deal of valuable information that encourages us to keep exploring.

Let's look at the construction of the organ itself. The brain consists of three main parts: the forebrain, the midbrain, and the hindbrain.

— The Three Major Parts of the Brain

The forebrain is the most recently evolved area of the brain. It consists of the cerebrum, thalamus, and hypothalamus (which is part of the limbic system).

The midbrain, which includes the uppermost portion of the brainstem, consists of the tectum and tegmentum. The midbrain is the smallest region of the brain and acts as a sort of *relay station* for auditory and visual information.

The hindbrain is the oldest part of the brain. It includes most of the brainstem, the cerebellum, the pons, and medulla. Often the midbrain, pons, and medulla are referred to together as the brainstem.

— The Cerebrum

The cerebrum or cortex (outer layer of the cerebrum) is the largest part of the human brain. Located in the forebrain, the cerebrum is associated with higher brain function such as thought and action. The cerebral cortex is divided into four sections called *lobes*: the frontal lobe, parietal lobe, occipital lobe, and temporal lobe. Here is a visual representation of the cortex:

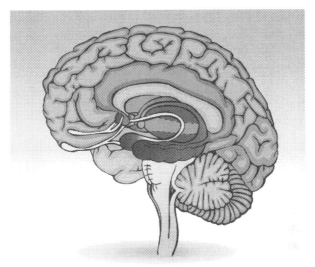

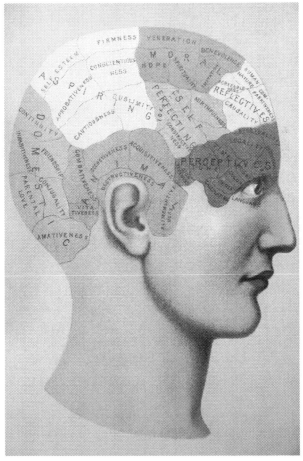

- **Frontal Lobe:**
  Associated with reasoning, planning, parts of speech, movement, emotions, and problem solving.

- **Parietal Lobe:**
  Associated with movement, orientation, recognition, perception of stimuli.

- **Occipital Lobe:**
  Associated with visual processing.

- **Temporal Lobe:**
  Associated with perception and recognition of auditory stimuli, memory, and speech.

— The Cerebellum

Also called "the little brain," the cerebellum is located in the hindbrain and is part of the brainstem. It is associated with regulation and coordination of movement, spatial perception, posture, and balance.

— The Limbic System

Often referred to as "the emotional brain," the limbic system is found deep within the cerebrum, above the brainstem. The limbic system is often called mammalian brain, because it is most highly developed in mammals. This system contains the thalamus, hypothalamus, amygdala, and hippocampus. The limbic system helps to maintain homeostasis, maintaining a stable environment in the body for survival. It regulates body temperature, blood pressure, blood sugar, heart rate, sexual desire. The limbic system is also involved with emotional response.

— Brain Stem

The brain stem is located underneath the limbic system. It is the oldest and the deepest area of the brain, having evolved more than five hundred million years ago—before the appearance of mammals. Many scientists refer to it as the "reptilian brain," because it looks like the entire brain of a reptile. This structure is responsible for basic vital life functions, such as breathing, heartbeat, and blood pressure. It is also called the survival center.

The problems with aging brains, forgetfulness, the feeling of brain fog, and learning difficulties are associated with the cerebral cortex and hippocampus (The brain receives information and organizes that information. Finally, it presents the information to guide our actions and behavior. Some information is saved in a "storage room" for future use. This information-processing center is the cerebral cortex. As Dr. Katz and Rubins put it,

> *The cortex is the part of the brain that is responsible for our unique human abilities of memory, language, and abstract thought. The hippocampus coordinates incoming sensory information from the cortex and organizes it into memories. The wiring of the cortex and hippocampus is designed to form links (or associations) between different sensory representations of the same object, event, or behavior. (Katz and Rubins, 1999, 46)*

> *(Lawrence C. Katz, Ph.D.,1956-2995, Neuroscientist, professor of neurobiology and pioneering researcher at Duke University Medical Center.)*

— Brain Hemispheres

The brain is divided into two halves, the left brain or hemisphere and the right brain or hemisphere. Both hemispheres are involved in higher cognitive functioning, with each half of the brain specialized in a complementary way for different modes of thinking, both highly complex. Strangely enough, the left brain controls the right side of the body and the right brain controls the left side of the body. That is why when you see a stroke patient who has one side paralyzed, the damage is found in the opposite side of the brain. The two sides of the brain are similar in shape, but they each handle different intellectual activities in addition to the different physical activities.

For a long time, the left-brain hemisphere was thought of as the most important side, whereas the right-brain hemisphere was considered somewhat less important. But the reality is that both sides of our brains are equally important. Most people have dominance on one side or the other. They are either left-brain dominant, or right-brain dominant. Few people have both sides of the brain with equal strength. Some people know they have a dominant side and pay special attention to strengthening both sides of their brains. Those who pay attention to strengthening both sides are considered really smart and intelligent. It seems these people, who work on enhancing both sides are less easily confused, have less sickness and fewer problems in their lives. Also, these people have a better chance to succeed in things they want to do, the goals they want to achieve, the relationships they want to maintain, and the business they want to pursue.

Functionality and Characteristics Attributed to the *Left Brain*

- **Verbal:** We can use words to name and express things clearly and to process language into meaningful communication.

- **Analytical:** We can figure out things in a step-by-step manner. We analyze things and then put things together in a reasonable way.

- **Symbolic**: We can use symbols to stand for something.

- **Abstract:** We are able to describe a whole story in a few paragraphs.

- **Temporal:** We can keep track of time, agendas, and activities in a timely and efficient way.

- **Sequential:** We can deal with events sequentially, organize information in a set order

- **Compositional:** We can write articles in scientific way.

- **Rational:** We can draw conclusions based on reason and fact.

- **Logical:** We can draw conclusions by making inferences from what is known.

- **Linear:** We can think of things as linked ideas, one thought leading to the next.

- **Computational:** We can use mathematics and arithmetic to count abstract amounts.

- **Practical:** We can do and make things that are useful and utilitarian in the moment.

- **Concrete:** We can think of things as explicit, precise units.

Functionality and Characteristics Attributed to the *Right Brain*

- **Nonverbal:** We can respond to tones, sounds, body language, and touch.

- **Synthetic:** We can put separate things together to form a whole.

- **Concrete:** We can relate to things as they are, in the present moment.

- **Non-temporal:** We can ignore or transcend time and agendas.

- **Analogical:** We can perceive likenesses and virtual and metaphoric relationships.

- **Visual/Spatial:** We perceive shapes and patterns, can intuitively estimate sizes and distances, imagine real things in a mental sphere.

- **Intuitive:** We can make leaps of insight, often based on feelings and intuition.

- **Holistic:** We can see the big picture of things, seeing overall relationship, patterns, structures.

- **Spontaneous:** We can handle things spontaneously, casually, informally, according to the needs of the moment.

- **Creative:** We are able to come up with new ideas and theories based on our experience and learning

- **Metaphoric:** Our ideas are symbolic, representational.

From the above list, it appears the logical, objective left brain fits more with Western philosophy or culture, whereas the intuitive, subjective right brain fits more with Eastern philosophy or culture. Certainly, there are many great scientists and inventors in the United States, and more than enough artists and crafts people in China. But, from Daoist philosophy and yin and yang theory, there is no absolute category for either one. Yin and yang can change, transform, and communicate. Yin and yang supplement and assist each other. They complement, support, and rely on each other. The brain is the same way. Its function can change and transform. The two sides of the brain can assist, complement, support, and rely on each other. The weaker side of your brain can be strengthened by proper training. This is referred to as *neuroplasticity*. In fact, if you have a business, you need to develop both sides of your brain, because any good or successful business requires both sides of the brain to function in harmonious way.

What I call the "Eastern Brain" refers to the typical Asian way of doing or processing things, or generally coming from Eastern philosophy. It may not refer to a Westernized Asian person's way of approaching things, just as what I call "Western Brain" does not refer to the way every American or person from the West perceives and proceeds. Many Asians have assimilated to Western cultural ideas very successfully, and many Westerners have adopted Asian cultural ideas with aplomb as well. It is certainly clear from my recent visits to China that the Chinese culture is becoming Westernized in some areas, just as we see evidence of Asian cultural influences here in the U.S. Perhaps we are moving toward a global, balanced brain? We'll see.

— Eastern and Western Brains

Here are some examples of the behavioral differences between the so-called Western and Eastern brains. These examples are meant to illustrate rather than be definitive. And again, they are not meant to imply that one is better than another, nor that all people of a particular race or culture exhibit these same qualities. There are no absolutes.

- **Cooking**

   The traditional Western style of cooking is to follow a recipe that lists the exact ingredients, quantities, cooking method, temperature, special equipment needed, and so on. Even when trying to learn from friends or family, most people ask, "Would you please give me the recipe?" Whereas the Asian style of cooking uses general varieties and amounts of ingredients such as salt, pepper, soy sauce, vinegar, ginger, garlic, and hot pepper to create many dishes. When trying to learn a new dish from friends or family, they get the main ingredients and general instructions from conversation and then follow their own taste for the specifics.

- **Traveling or Vacationing**

   Many Western travelers like to plan far in advance, scheduling flights, booking hotels, buying tickets for attractions, and making restaurant reservations well ahead of embarking on their trips. Many Asian travelers go places when they feel like it, mapping the route as they go, and staying at whatever hotel they find along the way. However, as the wealthy middle class continues to grow in China, and as time becomes scarcer with work schedules, their approach to making holiday plans will likely become more Westernized.

- **Disease and Healing**

   In the West, most disease diagnosis involves conducting tests on the patient to isolate the cause, interpreting the results, and making treatment recommendations aimed at specific symptoms. The measurement of results of healing are based on technology findings or lab test findings. The Eastern approach views disease as an imbalance and stagnation of energy flow; healing work focuses on correcting the root of the problem and allowing the person to heal him or herself; the measurement of results of healing are based on what the person reports about their overall feeling, as well as the healer's evaluation of the patient. Therefore, the quality of the practitioner is very important.

- **Values**
  Traditional Western values, in general, tend to lean very much toward materialism. This is related to the capitalist economic system. Traditional Eastern values often lean more toward the value of family life, harmony, a search for balance in one's life, and personal well-being. Today, many people, from the East and West, are blending both traditions, in a search for the best of both.

- **Regulations**
  Westerners follow rules very well; yes means yes and no means no. Whereas, in the East, many people follow the rules well only to certain degree. Sometimes, to some people, yes can change to no, and no can change to yes depending on the situation. I call this "elasticity."

- **Working**
  In the West, in many cases the company is the main structure for conducting business, often with a management team led by a CEO, a detailed organizational structure, modern IT systems and controls for achieving the firm's objectives. The ownership of the company is often through its shareholders, if the company is public. Whereas many companies in the East are still owned and run by a patriarch and his family. This again is changing as more companies go public in Asia. However, in the West, it is clear that separating ownership from management does not always lead to the best decisions being made for the company or its shareholders. There is something to be said for Western management behaving more like owners of a company rather than as temporary tenants. Eastern workers, however, seem more loyal to the company and more willing to work hard. This may have something to do with the competition and huge population.

- **Lifestyle and Financial Planning**
  Most people in the West plan ahead for retirement, whereas, in traditional Eastern culture, the tendency is to save money for the

children until they are well established. As long as they're not, the family may continue to support them. I have seen many Asians who saved money their whole lives while maintaining poor life styles, but nonetheless left money to their children when they died. Fortunately, in most Asian families, the children also take care of their parents when the parents are older, disabled or have some medical issue that requires assistance.

- **Dealing with People**
Westerners often express things directly, making their viewpoint clear; whereas in the East, people express things less straightforwardly. Sometimes you even might have to guess what the speaker really means. This can sometimes causes confusion and misunderstanding.

- **Activities**
Popular Western culture encourages thrill-seeking behavior as people seek excitement and that rush of adrenaline; whereas in Eastern cultures, contemplative behavior, finding peace, tranquility and beauty in quiet, stillness, and calm continues to be valued.

Since the world is changing, tradition and culture everywhere is also changing. People are getting smarter and trying to learn whatever is good for their lives. Living in New England for over twenty years, I still see many people living their lives in a traditional way. And others are trying to make their lives better with a balance of tradition and change.

A long-term patient of mine named John, used to be so stubborn and stiff in his ways. He is a brilliant man and very analytical with everything. Working with him was a challenge for me. I was trying to help him with his many physical ailments, and also trying to educate him about Daoist philosophy, which could offer him new skills for stress management and relaxation exercises. I also gave him some extra homework to help him to balance both sides of his brain. Because of his stubbornness and highly stressed personality, he was suffering with serious heart disease and hypertension. In Chinese medicine, the mind is closely related to heart energy. This explains why so many people with long-term stress are prone to heart disease and heart attacks. After working with him for a year using multiple approaches, his heart condition improved, his attitude improved, and he became much more relaxed and easy going. He was finally able to see things from multiple angles. Perhaps the biggest highlight was that his relationship with his family improved.

Research done by Dr. Robert Ornstein (University of California) found that the left brain handles these mental activities:

- Mathematics
- Language
- Logic
- Analysis
- Writing
- And other similar activities

The right side brain handles different activities:

- Imagination
- Color
- Music
- Rhythm
- Daydreaming
- And other similar activities

Ornstein also found that people who had been trained to use one side of their brain more or less exclusively were relatively unable to use the other side, both in general and in specific situations where activities were related to the other side of the brain. He also found that when the "weaker" of the two hemispheres was stimulated and encouraged to work in cooperation with the stronger side, the result was a great increase in overall ability and effectiveness. From Make the Most of Your Mind by Tony Buzan

Most of us were trained in traditional thinking that believes that strong left-brainers do well with reading, writing, arithmetic; and right-brainers will do well in art, music, spatial relationships, etc. This kind of thinking uses old findings and theories to put people into a box, saying that the person who has a strong right brain has less chance of success in science and business; whereas the person who has a strong left brain has less chance of success when using common sense and intuition. But this is really too simplistic; our brains are not completely separated. The right brain is just as important as the left brain for proper functioning in each individual.

Since our two brains are connected through the corpus callosum, a large bundle of nerve fibers cross-connecting the two cerebral hemispheres, the two brains can cooperate to do similar work, and the weak brain can become stronger through training. The potential is there that if we train ourselves to work with both sides of the brain, and give them enough stimulation, we can achieve a great deal, no matter which side of the brain may be stronger.

This explains why the brain will benefit from tai chi practice and learning. The 360-degree movements in space force your right and left hemispheres to communicate back and forth, trading off dominance in a continuous, integrated exercising of the brain and body. We will discuss this in detail later.

— Brain Aging and Brain Anti-Aging

The brain is the most important and complex organ in the human body. This doesn't mean that other organs are not important. The brain does magical work in our daily lives and throughout our lifetime. It regulates and assists us with our health, healing, learning, creativity, emotions, senses, and so much more. This is why so many scientists spend whole lifetimes sometimes studying the brain and "mind power." In addition, many holistic health practitioners use their knowledge and experience with the brain, mind, and awareness to guide patients to heal themselves in their healing work. In my practice with natural healing and natural medicine, I have seen many miracles; it is as if anything is possible if you put enough of your effort, your intent, your focus, your beliefs, your imagination, and your energy into the work. When cancer heals, it particularly shows the meaning and the value of mind-body healing.

The brain is composed of some one hundred billion cells called neurons. The neuron, unlike other cells, has many arms or branches like an octopus. These millions of branches are like tentacles radiating in all directions. They are called dendrites. Each of these dendrites has thousands of tiny protuberances, much like the suction pads on the tentacles of the octopus, but protruding from all sides. These form communication pathways between nerve cells that form the basis of learning and memory. We have always believed that intelligence is related to the number of brain cells, and poor memory was due to the loss of brain cells. We were also taught that brain cells could not be replaced.

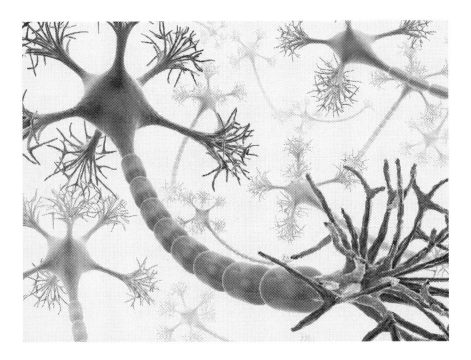

Scientists have now determined that the adult brain not only can grow new cells, but can also sprout new dendrites. Scientists know now that it is not the number of the brain cells that determines a person's intelligence, but rather that intelligence is associated with the protuberances on the brain cells' tentacles. Crossing the protuberances of each brain cell, electrochemical impulses form patterns with individual cells and groups. To put it another way, it is like a human social network: if you know one person, you may learn things from that one person; if you know many different people and communicate with them all, you may learn many different things. These dendrites on the nerve cells receive and process information from other nerve cells, thus forming the basis of memory. When our minds are not used, or not adequately challenged, we risk losing a great deal of our potential brain power. If the dendrites don't communicate regularly, they can atrophy. This reduces the ability to put new information into memory, and makes it difficult to retrieve old information. This also reduces other brain functioning such as cognitive ability, spatial orientation, and logical ability.

For as long as I can remember, it has been assumed that the brain declines with age. This decline included memory, attention span, numerical ability, creativity, alertness, learning ability, and language. It's been so widely believed that we've all heard the expression "you can't teach an old dog new tricks." But we were wrong. New data indicates that you *can* teach an old dog new tricks—*if* the old dog is willing to learn and the trainer is willing to train. It is true that our bodies degenerate with age. But the brain is not the same; this mysterious organ does not get old side-by-side with the body. New findings from science show that if the brain is consistently stimulated, no matter at what age, the brain can remain young and healthy; it doesn't matter if you are forty or seventy. With stimulation of the brain through all kinds of activities, the brain will generate new connections far more rapidly, on average, than it will lose brain cells. Keep this in mind: it's the connections and the communication between the brain cells that keeps our brains young, keeps our memory working, makes our brains function well, and keeps us intelligent and creative. Many experts agree that the adult brain can *improve* with age, and this has been demonstrated through scientific study.

The human brain is a biological supercomputer. Even though we have learned a great deal of information about the brain to date, there is so much more for us to explore.

How Tai Chi and Qi Gong Prevent Brain Aging and Memory Loss

As we age, our bodies slow down, and we tend to become forgetful. The good news is that research has shown that if we manage our daily activities using daily physical exercise, and other skill practice, we can maintain and even restore our memory function and learning ability. I have been experimenting with this my whole life in an effort to support my health, my learning, my overall improvement, and my memory. My goal is to avoid dementia and physical disability, and be able to enjoy my life for as long as I can. There is also clinical science to support what my hypothesis tells me is possible.

Practicing tai chi, qi gong and other body movement exercises is very effective to preventing human aging and brain aging. Over thousands of years, there is visible evidence of people affecting the quality of their own health and well-being, increasing their longevity, stamina, and cognitive powers. History teaches us that we need to let go of things without value, and to keep things that are valuable. From thousands of years of experience, the people in China know why they need to do certain things, and they know how to do them. Whereas in the West, people seem to require a scientific explanation for all the why and how questions. For instance, I would hazard a guess that many, if not most people living a Daoist lifestyle in China, would be hard put to explain it, if you asked them about the Dao. Some of them probably don't even know what the Dao is. Recently more and more research has been done to place it on a scientific level, so perhaps people are becoming better educated about it, but they used it successfully even before.

Using tai chi and qi gong to prevent brain aging is presented here from my own experience, including the changing behavior and attitudes seen in my students, as well as the observations of many masters. I have summarized this hypothesis this way:

1. *Lifelong Learning*

Human learning should never stop. I always tell my family, and I cover it in my lectures and speaking, that the day you stop learning is the day you stop living. Learning is a big part of healing; healing is a big part of learning. Tai chi involves learning big time. When you start to learn things you don't know, you start to shift your focus onto new knowledge, new approaches, new movement, and a new life style. Tai chi learning is continuous and multileveled in skill, depth, and meaning. Through continuous learning and practice, you will get the meaningful part—the true nature of tai chi. If you are just starting as a beginner, you will feel good immediately, from the exercised practice of relaxation. If you are an advanced student, you will feel good continuously, from the sustained practice of energy fluidity. Either way, you get benefits. Even people who do it incorrectly still get benefits. As you practice for more than a year or two, your tai chi form will become more graceful and beautiful, and you will feel like you are dancing in the clouds. This gives you an added feeling of accomplishment and satisfaction. Learning tai chi is challenging, but the challenge will lead to building a flexible brain that will support you as you age.

Any kind of challenge is a type of stimulation to our brains. Without challenge, we would never be able to invent things; without challenge, our living would not advance. If we rely on a calculator all the time, soon we can't calculate easy equations anymore. If we store every phone number in our cell phone contacts list, or computer, we'll never be able to remember any of those phone numbers anymore. In one scientific study on aging and the brain, scientists confirmed that *any* intellectually challenging activity and *any* mildly complex movement activity stimulates dendrites to grow, and this adds more connections in the brain's neural pathways.

When you work on learning tai chi or qi gong, it is like you are shifting gears into a positive energy drive. The more positive energy you have, the more improvement you will have in all aspects of your life and being. Improvement is always a good thing; this is how our lives get better and better each year. The positive energy also goes to your brain, and therefore all your body's parts function better.

Just as there are two sides of the brain, there are two types of thought: conscious and unconscious. Conscious thought involves your awareness of the day, your plans for the day, plans for work or travel, your pleasures, and your peeves. You can logically rearrange, discuss, and guide your behavior according to your needs. Unconscious thoughts, on the other hand, are more spontaneously occurring and out of your intentional control, such as holding a cup, saying goodnight to your spouse, your heart beating fast when you are nervous. Observing tai chi practitioners, it seems that conscious thought is enhanced, empowering you to be more in tune with your daily experiences.

2. A Break in Your Routine

We grow up with certain fixed routines and most of us don't want to change these routines. Such routines may include our diets, activities, thought processes, opinions, and lifestyles. We don't like to do something if we are not familiar with it. While on a hiking trip with my sister and my husband in Acadia National Park, we got disoriented in the woods. My sister and I wanted to explore for a way out, but my husband insisted that we go back the same way to get out. Seeing his anxiety, I almost gave up and agreed to go back same way. Suddenly my sister found a new path. It guided us onto another main path, and we found our way back on track. She broke the routine and helped us find our way.

Routines can be brain deadening. When something unusual happens and gets us out of our routine, we get anxious; we sometimes don't know what to do. We feel like our brains are not working. Just think, many of us go to work every day, come home, eat, sleep, go to work the next day—our brains are programmed in such a way that we don't even have to think any more. Our brain cells lose communication opportunities, certain neural pathways shut down. *Breaking the routine is a brain fitness workout.* This allows new activities for the brain and encourages brain cells to communicate, opening new neural pathways. Watching TV is another brain killing activity; this doesn't mean we need to give up on TV. I always like to watch the news and some nature programs and other educational programs. Research has shown that during TV watching, the brain is less active, even less active than during sleep! When you are watching TV, your brain is passive—or active in a passive way. Some TV program can even traumatize the brain, which can make us unable to view things as a whole. If you know how to balance your life, you will be careful to watch TV wisely, and add other brain fitness exercises into your life. Think for a moment: how many smart "couch potatoes" are there? (I don't mean people who watch TV are all couch potatoes).

Tai chi exercise and learning is not familiar to the majority of Americans. We did not grow up with slow-motion exercises; we like fast and vigorous; we like *pain*. We often hear "No pain, no gain." This is not an entirely accurate statement. In our early years, we struggled for everything; we suffered a lot; we had a lot of pain before we could gain. But now it is different, we don't have to suffer too much in order to gain. There has been so much change in our lives, our health, our society, our government, our technology, our earth, our lifestyle, our science, and more. That old statement also needs to change. Our needs are beyond surviving and just making a living. Our physical burdens have shifted to mental burdens. We need tools to help us to relieve the mental burdens. In other words, even exercise in this modern lifestyle should be balanced—fast *and* slow movements. The yin energy (receptive, slow) and the yang energy (active, fast) should be evident everywhere to keep our lives balanced. Many of our problems are caused by the imbalance of yin and yang. However, it is true that hard work, smart learning, and dedication can lead you to success.

Once you open your mind, you can purposely derail your routine and adjust your old habits. You can build brain cells by choosing to experience a totally new concept, a new philosophy, a new way of life, a new journey. Your brain cells will have to branch out to make new connections with other brain cells.

I keep saying that tai chi is a journey. That's because you are always learning new things from tai chi practice, acquiring new knowledge, finding new feelings, making new movements or understanding old movements more deeply, forging new friendships, and building new energy. Tai chi opens your mind and, along with it, a pathway to a new way of seeing things. On the practical side, it helps you to multitask in a way you may have never thought possible. It got my sister and my husband and me out of the woods.

3. Better, Deeper Sleep

We know that sleeping disorders can accelerate aging, especially brain aging. When you look at a person with a sleeping problem, the first thing you notice is that she or he looks tired. The next thing you notice is the speech is slow. This indicates that the brain language center is sluggish, less active. The same is true for other parts of the brain. We have all had the experience that if we don't sleep well the previous night, we notice that our minds are not clear, our memory is not sharp, and we cannot concentrate. Sleep-deprived, your brain has less ability to store new information, and less ability to retrieve the old information. In medical school, one of my most drastic problems was a sleeping disorder. This couldn't have helped my memory problems. The day I graduated, I said to myself, *I never want to go back to school again*, even though I hadn't done poorly at all.

Many of my patients who have sleeping problems tell me, "My brain is in a fog," or they'll say, "I can't remember things …" If a person has had a long-term sleeping disorder, you can see that she looks older than her actual age. A good night's sleep is also an important part of healing in dealing with many illnesses. Just think about a machine, if used nonstop, the machine soon breaks down.

With regular practice of tai chi and qi gong, your neurochemicals become balanced, your body's electricity regulated, your sleeping becomes regulated, your brain exhaustion is relieved, brain alertness restored. Now, brain healing can begin. And so it does.

4. Increased Oxygen

I mention oxygen so many times in my lectures, speeches, classes, trainings, short talks, long talks, and conversations, because it is so important to life and health. The brain, although only about 2 percent of your body weight, consumes roughly 20 percent of the oxygen you breathe in! When the brain is nurtured with adequate oxygen, it helps to bring better function to the breathing center and vascular center. And vice versa. If you have problems with your heart and lungs that affect your oxygen level, it will also affect the oxygen level in your brain. Cognitive power declines when there is a decreased supply of oxygen to the brain.

When I see a person yawn too many times, I tease him, "You need more oxygen"; when I see a person who sleeps too much, I say, "You need more oxygen"; when I see a person driving and feeling sleepy, I say, "You need more oxygen"; when I see a person feeling tired, I say, "You need more oxygen." Oh boy, if your energy is flagging, you better not be near me! I feel like I am the mother of all nagging.

As we know, the brain must consume oxygen to be able to function. It is the lungs that help us to get oxygen through the breath. If your brain lacks oxygen for six to nine minutes, your brain can be damaged. If you lack oxygen for twenty minutes, you will die. If your body lacks food for fifteen days, you may still live. The oxygen to our brain is very important. If your brain has enough oxygen, you are most likely alert; if your brain lacks oxygen, you feel tired, lethargic, overcome by the old mind fog. You will also notice, when you are tired or feel sleepy, you feel a little more clear after a big yawn. Yawning is the deepest breath we can take; we do it to get oxygen to our tired brains. One of the most important parts of preventing brain aging is getting enough oxygen to it.

Practicing qigong and tai chi involves deep breathing, which helps to bring more oxygen to your body and your brain; you will notice the change in your overall feeling. You will feel less cloudy, fresher, more alert, and more energetic.

5. *Unique Tai Chi Movement Sequences*

Tai chi movements are not like any other exercise. The special, choreographed movements are circular, and in constant motion. Many gestures cross the body from left to right, from upward to downward, and from right diagonal to left diagonal. The footwork is also slow, on the diagonal, well controlled, and with multiple changing stances. Through the controlled, slow, smooth, multidimensional—in spatial dimension and internal dimension—whole body movements, you learn to be aware of your body. You become aware of your tension, your balance, your energy, your emotional stability, and your visual surroundings. You pay attention to your energy center and self-correct your posture. You pay attention to know if you are off-center, or you lose your balance. You move with your intention; you move your body while your mind experiences calm and peace.

During the tai chi movement, you get sensory stimulation, motor stimulation, spatial orientation stimulation, , forebrain and hindbrain stimulation, left-brain and right-brain stimulation, balance and equilibration stimulation, and cross-brain stimulation. Therefore, the whole brain is stimulated. Tai chi movements are very good brain fitness exercises. We use aerobic exercise to increase our heart rate and to promote better circulation; we also need brain fitness exercise to improve our brain function and learning abilities. Western science has confirmed that movement is crucial to brain health, and definitely affects cognitive change. Eastern practitioners of tai chi knew it all along. A later chapter will teach you some total body exercises and qi gong movements you can try out for yourself.

Evidence shows that movement is also crucial to every other brain function, including memory, emotion, language, learning, and more. After you have learned some qi gong later in the book, try if for three to five minutes when you are tired after working or writing a paper for a while and your brain can't seem to think anymore. You will realize you will be able to return to work refreshed, able to put more words on the paper. What is happening there? As we know, our "higher" brain functions evolved from basic mobility functions, and they still depend on them. Any immobile or sedentary lifestyle is prone to affect brain aging—too much TV or any other couch-potato, "brain dead" activity.

The well known kinesiology and learning researcher Dr. Paul Dennison, along with his wife, movement educator Gail Dennison, have developed a movement program that has been proven to exercise the brain, they call it

Brain Gym. Brain Gym, is a movement-based technique to enhance learning ability for children with learning difficulties in conventional settings. As adults age, our learning styles tend to mimic that of these kinds of children. We do not learn as quickly or as well as younger people. The information takes longer to put into memory storage, and it takes longer to learn new things. Studies have shown that we shift from visual and auditory learners to *kinesthetic* learners. That is, we don't absorb so much from reading or listening as we once did; we need to learn by doing. Above and beyond learning style, Brain Gym has helped to establish even stronger links between certain kinds of movement techniques and enhancing brain function in general. The exercise movements and qi gong described in this book are designed to help adults achieve maximum learning and delay the brain aging process. See later chapter for details.

I have a friend named Nancy. Nancy's husband has several systems hooked into the television, and therefore needs several different remotes. In order to watch TV, she has to use several buttons on each remote to watch TV. Even though her husband has taught her several times, she still cannot find the right button to turn on the TV. Finally, she just bought another TV with only one remote. Many older people have trouble using multi-system entertainment centers. On the other hand, one of my tai chi students studied piano at the age of fifty-eight. She told me that her piano teacher was amazed at her ability to learn the piano. My own experience was learning cello—I didn't start until I was forty-nine. I was skeptical, myself! But now I realize I can learn; and I even improved. It is rewarding to see the improvement.

With certain body movements to simulate neural pathways, you enable nerve cells to communicate with each other, and create more activity in the brain network. Therefore, the participant feels more alert and can more easily put memory into storage, and later retrieve the information. That is why we say tai chi enhances learning ability.

Tai chi and qi gong exercise balances both sides of the brain by encouraging cross connections with information between left and right brain. With this special training, our dominant side can become more cooperative with the other, fostering a greater balance between the two sides. This hemispheric balance helps you to develop well-balanced cognitive, communication, and social skills. Once your brain is more balanced, you may even be more pleasant with your partner or companion, more easy going, better able to multitask, more even-tempered, more able to learn new things, and less rigid or stubborn. These are some of the changes that I have observed first hand in many of my students.

The cross-brain movements create a sort of cross-brain training. The stimulation causes more communication to occur through synapses of the brain cells. This enhanced connection and communication between the brain cells keeps our brains young and our memory strong.

Science has also confirmed that tai chi improves the body's balance. The cerebellum controls balance, coordination, adjustment, and smoothing out of movement. Tai chi improves the cerebellum's function; therefore the benefits become evident in better coordination and balance.

Recent studies have shown that the cerebellum is not just related to movement, but also to cognition. If a person has injuries in the brain and cerebellum, there are studies that suggest a possibility for improvement from tai chi and qigong practice. Since tai chi improves cerebellum function, it is likely tai chi will improve both physical balance and cognitive skill, each an indicator of brain health. By rewiring the brain itself, not only can the brain learn new tricks, but it can also change its structure and function, even in old age. Tai chi is really a brain fitness regimen for adults.

6. *Balance and the Autonomic Nerve System (ANS)*

In the human body, all functions are controlled through the nervous system, all *organs* are controlled by the autonomic nerve system; many illnesses are caused by disorders of these systems. My main healing focus is to regulate the nervous system which made a big difference in my healing ability.

— Understanding the Nervous System

The brain is Communication Central for the computer-like nervous system, a network of special tissue that controls all the actions and reactions of the body's functioning parts. Like a computer, the nervous system has memory storage capabilities. The spinal cord is the conducting cable for the computer's input and output, and the nerve fibers are the circuits that supply input information to the cable and transmit output commands to muscles and organs. Our nervous system helps our bodies regulate and adapt to whatever changes occur in our environment.

Our nervous system has two main divisions: the central and the peripheral nervous systems. The central nervous system consists of the brain and the spinal cord. Linked to these are the cranial, spinal, and autonomic nerves, which, with their branches, constitute the peripheral nervous system.

Autonomic nerve impulses originate in the central nervous system and perform the most basic human functions automatically, without conscious intervention of higher brain centers. Autonomic nerve fibers exit from the central nervous system as part of other peripheral nerves but branch from them to form subsystems: the sympathetic, the parasympathetic, and the enteric nervous systems. The actions of the sympathetic and parasympathetic systems usually oppose each other. For example, sympathetic nerves cause arteries to contract, while parasympathetic nerves cause them to dilate. The sympathetic division typically functions in actions requiring quick responses. The parasympathetic division functions with actions that do not require immediate reaction. Consider sympathetic as "fight or flight" and parasympathetic as "rest and digest." Generally, these two systems should be seen as permanently modulating vital functions, in usually antagonistic fashion, to achieve homeostasis.

The sympathetic nervous system connects the internal organs to the brain via spinal nerves; it responds to stress by increasing heart rate and blood flow to the muscles and decreasing blood flow to the skin. The parasympathetic nervous system comprises the cranial nerves and the lower spinal nerves, which increase digestive secretions and slow the heartbeat. Both have sensory fibers that send feedback on the condition of internal organs back to the central nervous system, information that helps maintain homeostasis. The enteric system is a specialized subsystem of nerves embedded in the walls of the stomach and intestines—these control digestive movement and secretions.

The autonomic nerve system regulates the iris of the eye and the smooth-muscle action of the heart, blood vessels, glands, lungs, stomach, colon, bladder, and other visceral organs; it therefore affects heart rate, digestion, respiration, salivation, perspiration, pupils, urination, bowel movement, and sexual arousal—all responses that seem automatic and outside our conscious control. The autonomic system is influenced by the emotions, of course; for example, anger can cause your heart to race (heart rate), and fear can spoil your appetite (salivation) or shut your digestion right down.

Patients visit their doctors for unexplained symptoms; they are disappointed when doctors cannot find anything wrong and cannot help them. These unexplained ailments are most likely caused by disorders of the autonomic nervous system. When I correct the imbalance of an autonomic disorder, the symptoms diminish and the patient feels better. When they call me "miracle worker," I just tell them what I did. The autonomic nervous system has a close relation to the meridian system in Chinese medicine. I love working with the nerve systems, especially the autonomic nerve system (ANS), because people can feel the difference acutely.

— Sympathetic Nervous System (SNS):

SNS promotes a "fight or flight" response, corresponds with arousal and energy generation, and inhibits digestion. Here are a few specific actions the SNS is responsible for taking in your body:

- Diverts blood flow away from the gastrointestinal (GI) tract and skin via vasoconstriction.

- Blood flow to skeletal muscles and the lungs is not only maintained, but enhanced.

- Dilates bronchioles of the lung, which allows for greater alveolar oxygen exchange.

- Increases heart rate and the contractility of cardiac cells, thereby providing a mechanism for the enhanced blood flow to skeletal muscles.

- Dilates pupils and relaxes the ciliary muscle to the lens, allowing more light to enter the eye and distance vision.

- Provides vasodilation for the coronary vessels of the heart.

- Constricts all the intestinal sphincters and the urinary sphincter.

- Inhibits peristalsis (the movements of the bowels).

- Stimulates orgasm.

— Parasympathetic Nervous System (PNS)

PNS promotes a "rest and digest" response, promotes calming of the nerves to return to regular function, and enhances digestion. Here are some specific examples:

- Dilates blood vessels leading to the GI tract, increasing blood flow. This is important following the consumption of food, due to the greater metabolic demands placed on the body by the gut.

- Constriction of the bronchiolar diameter when the need for oxygen has diminished.

- Cardiac branches of the vagus and thoracic spinal accessory nerves to impart parasympathetic control of the heart or myocardium.

- During accommodation, the parasympathetic nervous system causes constriction of the pupil and contraction of the ciliary muscle to the lens, allowing for closer vision.

- Stimulates salivary gland secretion, and accelerates peristalsis, so, in keeping with the rest-and-digest functions, appropriate PNS activity mediates digestion of food and indirectly, the absorption of nutrients.

- Stimulates sexual arousal with involvement in the erection of genitals, via the pelvic splanchnic nerves.

The movements in tai chi and qi gong, as well as total body warm up exercises, involve wholesale twisting and turning of the body, loosening the spine and all of the vertebrae joints. This makes these paired nerves work in harmony, balancing the autonomic nervous system, and therefore maintaining homeostasis in the body and brain. Deep and slow breathing stimulate the respiratory and circulatory centers in the brain, helping to regulate autonomic function.

7. *Building Qi, Harmonizing Energy*

Qi is vital energy, or life force. It is the energy that underlies everything in the universe. *Qi* in the human body refers to the various types of bio-energy associated with human health and vitality. Changing *qi* in our body can affect our health and well-being. When you breathe, air enters the lungs. The lungs extract the external energy and blend it into the bloodstream, which is already carrying the internal energy extracted by the digestion of food and water. The resulting blend is the basis for human energy, which is related to metabolism and immune function. *Qi* is present internally and externally; it controls the function of all parts of the body. There are many different types of *qi*, which is discussed, in my first book, *Natural Healing with Qigong*.

Tai chi and qi gong strengthen all of the organs—kidneys, heart, liver, spleen, and lungs. In TCM, the "kidney" system is related to the brain, the "heart" system is related to *shen* (spirit) and also to the brain. The "liver" system is related to emotions and moods and is also associated with the brain. The "spleen" system is associated with digestion, absorption, metabolism, and blood—all bringing nutrients to the brain. The "lung" system controls *qi* intake and is also related to the brain. All of the organs are related to the brain; the body and the brain are connected. By exercising the brain, you help the body; by exercising the body, you help the brain.

Working with this *qi*, this energy in the body, is like working with an electric power plant. We use the electricity generated by the power plant to enable us to perform all kinds of functions. By elevating body energy with tai chi or qi gong, we can stimulate the brain and affect the brain chemicals. This kind of practice engages your attention, puts you into a state of calm, and raises your relaxation response. For centuries, Eastern philosophers have known the connection between our minds and our bodies; this is the basis of qi gong.

All three components of *qi* practice—mental focus, body movement, and breath—affect our brain. The mind focuses to help us memorize, whereas when the opposite is true, there will be a scattered memory, a scattered mind. Body movements, together with deep breathing, help the energy go through the body smoothly, finally reaching and passing through the brain. As deep breathing is stimulating the respiratory and circulatory centers in the brain, it also gathers our attention. The body becomes like a well-tuned, biological super computer, as the network and the electricity reach equilibrium.

With the tai chi workout, your energy starts moving in the body smoothly, your energy pathways are opened, your internal organs start to work harmoniously, and your mind and body start to work together. You are more adept, more open to learning, more willing to try, willing to experience, your brain cells start to communicate. Each new thing you do makes more connections among brain cells. This harmonious energy also promotes rapid healing for illness.

8. *Balancing the Emotions*

Both the right and the left frontal lobes are very important for the regulation of emotion. They are needed for making decisions in both the social and personal realms. Because tai chi stimulates the whole brain, coordinating the left and right brain and stimulating the crisscrossing of information between the left and the right brains, the upper and lower brains, it also balances the limbic system, the emotion center. Neurotransmitters start flowing smoothly between the synapses. After seeing the changes in the emotional state of many of my students, I was compelled to write *Tai Chi for Depression* several years ago. (it is available in my clinic).

Tai chi balances emotion also by developing self-awareness, focus, positive thinking, and building strong qi. Emotional balance is very important to prevent brain aging and provides a good physical and mental environment for learning. It helps to maintain and improve our ability to learn. Having balanced emotions enables you to be focused and pay attention to what you are doing. This helps both learning and memory. An impaired emotional state can reduce learning ability and make a person prone to memory loss.

Many people use medication to treat emotional problems, I disagree with this approach. People want an easy way and a shortcut for their health issues. They don't realize that many medications can cause memory loss, brain fog, and brain aging.

A friend of mine, Lisa, a very sweet and smart friend, is dealing with an emotional issue. She has been suffering with depression for a long time, and she is using medications. One of the issues I have noticed with her is that she has a hard time remembering things, especially appointments and dates. This became a problem for me as well when I made special arrangements to meet with her and she forgot that she was supposed to meet me.

9. *Involvement in Martial Arts*

We all understand that martial art practice is intended to make you strong and disciplined. Martial arts can give you mental power that helps you to achieve. In almost every form of tai chi, there is some martial arts relevance. People choose to practice tai chi for different reasons—to find the inner peace, for relief of stress, for flexibility, for healing, for longevity, for increasing energy and stamina, or for martial arts and self-defense. Tai chi originated as a martial art, and some movements are more pronounced in their martial aspect and can be used for self-defense. These martial arts movements make you feel stronger, more powerful, and more in control of yourself. They give you a solid, safe, stable, and determined feeling. They make you feel good and help you to believe in yourself, and that helps you to succeed in anything else you want to do. Whatever you do, you need to feel good about yourself; you cannot succeed if you don't feel good about yourself.

10. *The Right Music.*

Music is everywhere. We listen to music when we drive, walk, workout in the gym, sit in the doctor's or dentist's or holistic healing office, or even at home. Music is important in our lives. Certain music can have healing effects, while some loud, noisy music can cause heart disease and increased blood pressure. Some music can even make you more depressed and sad, and some music can make you anxious. Younger people like fast and stimulating music, older people and those with heart disease like slow and relaxing music. If you try to use rock and roll music for tai chi practice, it won't work. Science has fully demonstrated the effects music has on our brains and on our health. Many studies have even shown that certain music can reduce tension and enhance specific types of intelligence, such as verbal ability and spatial-temporal reasoning.

The music used in tai chi practice, in general, is very relaxing, calming, and tranquil. Adding music to tai chi and qi gong practice gives double benefits for well being. Using relaxing music helps you slow the movement down and make you more aware of your movement in space and yourself in the moment. If you try to use different music, the results of practice can be different.

11. *Responding to Relaxation*

I have seen so many patients who are loaded with stress. I cannot say that I don't have any stress, but I can say that tai chi and qi gong helps me to manage it well most of the time. In addition, it helps me remain focused on what I do. If you carry a lot of stress, you have less blood flowing in your muscles, your muscles are weakened (this can be proven with muscle-testing techniques), and you feel tired; even your brain is tired. You may recall when you were stressed, you could not think straight. With long term carrying stress, eventually your muscles will become degenerated, and you will feel pain all over your body. Your doctor then might give you a diagnosis of fibromyalgia. You may think that you have found the answer and the cure will follow just by being diagnosed with "Fibromyalgia", but you do not have the answer. You only have a name, a word that does not mean anything.

If I were to give the name, it would be "poor circulation, chronic inflammation and degeneration in the muscle tissue." I have treated many people with "fibromyalgia"; these people take many medications or painkillers, but still have the pain. Many of these people develop other problems from the side effects of their medications. We now understand that to help fibromyalgia, the first thing is to get your blood and energy moving.

There are many ailments related to stress or tension over long periods of time, such as insomnia, headache, heart disease, hypertension, cholesterol, GI problems, sexual dysfunction, back problems, neck problems, inability to focus, and more. In addition, stress causes distraction; you lose focus; you lose your normal sense of what life is supposed to be like.

One of the characteristics of tai chi and qi gong is meditation in motion, the best analgesic for all these symptoms. It relaxes you, and you start to feel that all the stress is melting away. Your body holds less tension; you feel calmer and more peaceful. The relaxation you get from tai chi or qi gong practice allows your energy to move smoothly through the body, your overwhelmed brain gets a rest, your muscles relax, your emotions settle down, and the tiredness disappears. Your yin-yang energy flow and balance is restored. Once your muscles are relaxed, more blood flows into the muscle tissue. Therefore, your muscles become strong (muscle-testing can help you to compare). You become more comfortable in your own skin, more aware of yourself in space and on the planet, and consequently, more aware of where you hold the tension or feel the weakness. Now you've got something tangible to work on, which then restores your sense of what life is suppose to be. Once you are more relaxed, you are more positive. Your positive state of mind can cause brain structure and function to change, to heal, and balance your neurotransmitter levels, which are the keys to maintaining mood and emotion. This positive cycle gives you a balanced life and better health.

12. Becoming Rooted

In a modern life style, our energy above the waist is high and scattered; we are distracted with so many activities and overwhelming information. We don't know how to focus or how to find what we are really attracted to. If you ask some college students—even ask a thirty-five-year-old—what they would like to do for a career, many of them don't know what they want to do or what really interests them. Some of them might just go for whatever job can make the most money. But, what if it turns out that they are not happy with the money-making job?

Tai chi and qi gong help you to feel rooted, stable, and focused—and to find your passion. This kind of practice helps you become more aware of your self and your spirit. It makes you more able to "listen to your heart." Tai chi guides you closer to nature, it helps you think and act more naturally, more authentically. The more you do things naturally, the more you understand universal energy and how it works. Doing things in a natural way is part of the brain's learning pattern, and getting away from technology sometimes can be a beneficial relief. The less involved with nature we become, the more troublesome issues we have to deal with. There is a saying, "Less is more," "Do less is doing more." Being in tune with nature, you cannot go wrong.

13. Touching

Sometimes we rub sore muscles when we feel discomfort. Sometimes we massage our temple areas when we get headaches. If we fall and hurt a foot or leg, we use our hands to press on the injured area. Sometimes, if you go to the doctor and tell her you have knee pain, within few minutes, the doctor is offering to give you a prescription for your pain without even touching your knee. How does that make you feel? If your child has a headache, the first thing you do is to touch his head to feel if he has fever. You then rub his head, trying to make him feel better. Why is that? It is because touching is an important part of healing. Why do we need hugs and kisses? Because the sensation we get from these hugs and kisses indicate friendship, love, closeness, and the feeling of being cared for.

Touching can bring special benefits to our body, mind, and brain. Neuroscientists can see the effect of touch on the brain using a functional MRI (fMRI). There is an increase in blood flow that is correlated with an increase in neuronal activity. Touch appears to affect multiple brain regions at conscious and unconscious levels. Touch has a wide impact on the brain, influencing our sensations, movements, thought processes, and capacity to learn new movements.

Some of the warm-up exercises for tai chi, and qigong itself, involve self-massage and acupressure. Through these kinds of sensory stimulations, not only do our brains get immediate benefit, but also our total awareness is heightened. Our bodies' acupressure points are stations on the energy map. You are delivering *qi* to these stations during self-massage and slow and rhythmic breathing.

14. *Group Energy*

One of the highlights of tai chi and qi gong are not only ways to exercise, but they also provide a nice social activity. Human beings have always enjoyed participating in group activities, functions, performances, and other social events. Human beings are social beings. In the United States, there are thousands of associations, professional societies, churches, study groups, and even street gangs. People seek others like themselves to do the things they enjoy, to enrich their lives and spirits. Social activity brings a learning experience with it; the more you interact with people, the more you learn. Animals are the same—a dog loves to be part of a pack. Scientists are finding from animal study that animals raised in an enriched environment had at least twice as many new brain cells in the region of memory and learning as the control group. The stimulation of their environment also provoked the development of new connections (synapses) *between* neurons. They also found that animals that live in an enriched environment live longer as well.

Scientific research has repeatedly proven that social deprivation has severe negative effects on overall cognitive ability. Not only that, social deprivation can cause depression, anxiety, and other serious illness. For many people, daily exercise involves each individual working by themselves, either on the treadmill, elliptical machine, weight lifting, or running. We really don't have to interact with anyone else. In the gym, we usually work on individual groups of muscles, to speed our heart rate, to raise our blood pressure, work up a sweat to get our metabolisms going, in hopes of losing some weight, gaining some muscle mass, and bringing more blood to our brain.

With tai chi and qi gong, it is different. With tai chi and qi gong, it is recommended that the exercise be done in a group (even though you sometimes need to practice by yourself). Group energy is important and very beneficial in tai chi and qi gong. Tai chi practice depends on a great deal of group energy, whether practicing in a classroom or outdoors. Group practice fosters discussion, friendship, social connection, group harmony, and all the positive benefits you might expect from group energy. Tai chi and qi gong also bring blood and oxygen to the brain, and stimulate the connections between brain cells. The combination of tai chi and group energy can only enhance these effects. It is no wonder they are so helpful in preventing memory loss and enhancing learning ability. People who come and participate in tai chi class at our school, feel happy, joyful, comfortable, and relaxed.

Students tend to do better when they practice together, because the energy of each individual affects the energy of others in the class. The more energy channels an individual is able to open, the better the results will be from the tai chi practice. When everyone's energy channels are open, the whole area is loaded with energy. You cannot see this, but you can feel it. In any kind of work, teamwork always brings the best results. The harmonious group energy makes you feel good for a long time afterward too.

This is what one of our participants said:

As a young man, I have been capable of running a marathon and riding my bicycle 100 miles. After I ran the Boston Marathon, I felt I made my way to the top of the mountain: I did something that most people will never be able to physically do, for whatever reasons those may be. Even though I was in good physical shape, after starting my journey with Tai Chi, I realized I had trouble coordinating my body in certain ways!

Since that short time ago and with much dedicated practice, I have improved those coordination skills tremendously. And I have humbly realized I am not at the top of the mountain, but only at the beginning of a path!

Tai Chi has not only helped me physically, but mentally and spiritually as well. I have been stuck in a dead-end retail environment for the past six years. Through the influence of coming to Tai Chi and Qi Gong classes, I am now going to school to be a holistic health counselor I believe my journey in Tai Chi so far has empowered me to utilize a part of myself that was just lying dormant.

Therefore, even as a young man, I can personally attest to the all-encompassing well-being benefits of this awesome exercise!

—Matt G

Other Tips for Brain Anti-Aging and Enhancing Learning Ability

— Exercise

Physical exercise and body movement is crucial. It doesn't matter what kind of exercise you start with, Eastern or Western; doing both is even better. Power walking is a great brain-fitness exercise. Walking with a friend and talking is very good for the brain; it adds that all-important social aspect. In a word, you just have to *move* your body. Qi gong is a great exercise to start with because it is low-impact, free of injury, and whole body. My most favorite exercise is "Therapeutic Qi Gong". (Therapeutic Qi Gong is a type of medical Qi Gong we offer in our school as well as training our instructors. It is sometimes called "Chinese Yoga".)

— Keep Learning:

Always try to think about ways you can improve yourself in all dimensions. You can learn a new language, learn to play chess or cards or knitting or the piano, make things with your hands, become skilled at fixing things, play a musical instrument, join a new organization, meet new people, and explore new vacation places.

— Read

We always tell kids to read more to make them smarter. As adults, we should do the same thing. My father always admonished me when I did not read the newspaper when I was young. In order to please him, I started to read it. He was right; by reading the newspaper, I did learn a lot. Reading is always good for our brains. Reading aloud is even better, because you also have the sound stimulating it.

— Memorize Numbers

Practice remembering different number sequences—phone numbers, house numbers, birthdays, anything with a number. If by now, you still don't remember your social security number, you are in trouble. You will have to watch out for dementia or Alzheimer's disease later in life. If you don't have a memory problem now, it doesn't mean you don't need to practice. The more you practice, the better it is for your brain's health. Start practicing right away and work on it every day. As they say, "Use it or lose it."

— Party and Socialize

As we discussed before, socializing is a type of learning experience, and a great brain exercise. It definitely enhances your brainpower and promotes the connections of brain cells. Not only are you exposed to learning new things in a different way, you are encountering different personalities, levels of intelligence, information, backgrounds, cultures, food and drink, clothes, energy, and lots more. It makes a big difference in your life if you participate in social activities. I used to focus only on my work, feeling that going to social events was wasting my time. I was wrong, because my old timer training did not help my brain. I don't know if you have had this experience (I have seen many): a great physician, but pretty dumb in other ways; or a very smart scientist but has a very poor life style. Now that I do participate, and even host social events, I find that I meet many different people, and have made a lot of new friends in my life. They are wonderful people to be with. Many of my students become my friends too. Life is just so much more colorful; my mind is busy, but not always with work. Almost all centenarians studied by science have had a strong social life—they tend to be outgoing, easy going, multitalented, and hard working. What more evidence do you need?

— Sing

Singing, either with a group or on your own, accompanied or unaccompanied, even doing karaoke, is an excellent brain exercise and *qi* practice. When you sing, there is a lot going on in your body and your brain: you have to remember the words and the melody, and you have to try to stay in tune. These multiple stimulations make more connections in your brain's nerve branches and synapses. Next, you need to take big breaths to sing and hold the sound. The deep breathing and sound vibration make a great *qi* practice. Sound has energy. The vibration and energy stimulate the brain like a wakeup call. Singing helps you to quickly move *qi* and build better stamina.

I suggest that you try this experiment when you are driving and feeling tired and sleepy. Just sing out loud and see what happens: suddenly your feel awake, alert, and you can keep your eyes open. That's because you are moving *qi*.

Too many of us are shy about singing in public. When we offered karaoke at our office party, most people said, "I don't sing," or even "You don't want to hear me singing." I had to keep telling them, "This is just for fun; it's not a competition!" Some people were willing to try, but others would not even pick up the microphone. My American husband used to get bothered at hearing my singing. He was not a big karaoke fan. So I stopped singing, for many years. After awhile, I realized I could not sing well anymore and felt somewhat depressed—something was missing in my life. When I went to visit China, I found out what it was. I went singing with my friends at a karaoke room; all of them sang better than me. And I used to be the best one! It was then that I realized: *It is the vibration energy I am missing.* That's when I decided to sing whenever I got chance—I would practice for my own health and have more fun in my life at the same time. Now, after many years of partying with karaoke, even my husband likes it! Another amazing part is that he has changed, of course in many good ways.

I suggest you start to sing, even if it's just in the car while you are driving—for fun, for energy, and for exercising your brain. And please visit www.karaokeeveryone.com. You won't be sorry.

— Be Present

Whatever you do, you should pay attention to it. Paying attention to what you are doing helps you to achieve better results. It helps you to avoid stress. If you have ten things to do, you should start one thing, focus on it, finish it; then you can start work on the next thing, focus on it, finish it, and so on. In this way, you will get much more accomplished. Any time you get distracted, you need to remind yourself to be present and pay attention to the task at hand. Ask yourself very often, "What am I doing now; where is my mind now?" This way you are able to get your thoughts back on track. Pay attention to where you are, who is around you, what subject is being discussed, and what is the goal of the task at hand. This helps to keep your brain-function more logical.

Chinese Medicine for Brain Health

Traditional Chinese Medicine (TCM) is a mind-body medicine, whole health medicine. The meridian system goes through all body parts, including the brain. By stimulating these energy pathways, the brain receives signals. It is like turning a switch on to make the connections better between nerve cells. People have told me that they feel more alert, and their brains are clearer. With the appropriate tune-up, your neurochemicals become balanced, and this helps to prevent brain aging and memory loss. Getting periodic care with TCM, you definitely have fewer physical complaints and fewer emotional complaints. With Chinese medicine care, it is always "two for price of one" because the practitioner always tries to treat your multiple ailments. This is unlike Western medicine, where we have to go to so many different specialists for what are really related ailments.

My worst experience was trying to make an appointment with an ENT, an ear, nose, and throat specialist. The receptionist told me that the next available opening was in five months. I said, "In five months, I might be dead." I was only partly kidding. She replied, "Do you want this appointment or not?" I took it, even though I was not pleased, but canceled several hours later. I felt if she could be that rude to me as a patient, then the office could probably not provide me with good healthcare. It felt like a machine shop that provided machinery service. So I did not get this appointment. I am still living after 3 years, no problem. I guess I didn't need a specialist after all. I am sure there are many good ones out there who are truly caring about their patients; you just have to find them. I guess if the receptionist knew I am an author and healer, she would not be rude. But, I may be wrong.

TCM offers a variety of treatment modalities that look at all your complaints as related—after all you are one person, with one body; your health should be treated as one whole.

— Acupuncture

Your meridian system is a big computer network. By stimulating certain points, it opens up the channels, and, therefore, balances the mind, and emotions. Acupuncture is a great way to keep your energy pathways open. There are many points related to your brain, even when just treating your body. Unblock the pathways and stimulate the brain,, that is what helps to balance brain chemicals.

— Chinese Massage (Tui Na)

Massage also gives sensory stimulation to the brain, as discussed previously in the touch section. Tui na is an excellent therapy to keep you happy and an ideal alternative if you are afraid of needles. Some people like tui na so much, they use it regularly as preventive medicine care. Periodic tui na helps you remain physically and mentally relaxed and emotionally balanced. You feel that you're getting true care with healing energy from the practitioner's hands.

If you can find a good and well-trained practitioner, Chinese message is a very pleasant treatment. We offer a tui na training program once a year at our clinic in Massachusetts. This training has provided many quality practitioners with useful knowledge and skills. Our patients are very happy with these practitioners.

One of my patients asked me if I am able to help children with emotional and learning disability. She told me that her daughter Mandy, age 14, had Asperger's syndrome with depression. Mandy was on heavy medication and suffered with depression, weight gain, inability to focus or do school work, anxiety, and anger issues. She could only read for a few minutes, and she had major social issues. I explained how natural medicine can help this condition, but I did not promise anything. She decided to make an appointment for her daughter with me.

When Mandy came to see me the first time, she did not look at me when she talked to me. She spoke to me with a tough tone, an upset attitude, and was very anxious, fidgeting throughout. She had no faith in herself and thought that she was stupid, fat, and that nobody liked her. I did a meridian examination of her body and found that her body had blockages in many areas. She argued with me, disagreeing with my professional recommendations.

I explained in a calm tone how she could be helped with natural medicine and exercise, and finally, she was open to the treatment. I did a combination of tui na, acupressure, and some qigong massage. She became a lot calmer right after the treatment. I then prescribed and taught her three exercises and some simple qigong, which were targeted to her symptoms. I asked her to make sure to do them at home and also gave some other homework, including a change in diet and some mental exercises.

When she came for second visit, she was a different person. She had done the homework I gave her that first visit, and she had changed her diet. She looked much calmer and spoke to me with a sweet smile, agreeing with my recommendations. When I checked her body meridians, her blockages were much better.

After five visits, she had lost weight, could read for a much longer period of time, was doing her homework by herself, and she mentioned that her depression was gone. The whole family was very happy with her progress. But I knew she still had ways to go. As I mentioned before—learning should never stop.

Another patient, Dorothy, was diagnosed with dementia. She forgot names quite often, didn't remember events from the day before, and could not remember some commonly used words. Her husband, Mark, was frustrated. They came to me, and Dorothy was under my care for several months. From the treatments and exercises I prescribed to her, she was able to make a big difference in her language and memory. Mark could not believe it. Loss of memory in the aging process is normal, but we can certainly decelerate this with natural therapy. From Dorothy's case, we know that anything is possible, including delaying the damage of early aging.

Two patients sent me these testimonials:

Dear Chinese Medicine for Health,

THANK YOU. I have just come home from a treatment today, and I just feel simply amazing. The massage and the acupuncture treatments made me feel like I had lost about 10 pounds, and I hit the gym after and had the best workout I've had in about a year. No pain in my knees or shoulders when I lifted or used the elliptical. So, thank you, thank you, thank you—and so far, I have called a few more of my friends and will hopefully be bringing them with me to see just how WONDERFUL you are.

—Anna H., Cape Cod, MA

Dear Dr. Kuhn,

I just wanted to share with you that I woke up this morning feeling alert and glad to be alive. (I don't often wake up that way.) I feel wonderful, have energy I haven't had in a long time, and best of all, have hope. Thank you so much. I love being alive again! All the best to you!"

—Jennie K., NY

The Difference between Tai Chi and Qi Gong

"What is the difference between tai chi and qi gong?" This is a question I often hear from my students and people attending my workshops. In the United States, more people know about tai chi than qi gong. They don't associate the two. They see them as individual and separate Chinese exercises. In reality, both tai chi and qi gong are internal energy workouts. They are both a part of the same energy science. Tai chi has a history of over four hundred years, whereas qigong has a history of over four thousand years. Qi gong is clearly the father of tai chi.

Tai chi is a type of qi gong, a higher-level qi gong that requires many years to learn well. Tai chi requires motor skill and coordination. Qigong requires no particular skill. Generally speaking, tai chi is much more challenging, is a deeper workout, and ultimately, more fun than qi gong. There are five main styles of tai chi: Yang, Chen, Wu', Wu, and Sun. They look different from each other, and the workouts are done differently, but they all have the same basic principle. Chen style is the oldest, and Yang style is the easiest. The most popular styles in China and the United States are the easier Yang style, followed by the Wu style, and then the Chen style. The most powerful and the closest to martial arts is, first, the Chen style, and then the Wu style. Besides being the oldest, Chen style is the most difficult form. All the tai chi forms are, in some part, a qi gong workout.

Qi gong is easier than tai chi. It also has many different forms from which to choose. Some of them can be more difficult than others. Some people think qi gong is too boring and not challenging enough. This is because they don't really know qi gong well and haven't practiced it properly. If you practice qi gong right, it is not boring at all.

There was one type of qi gong that I used to practice that was very hard, and so I chose not to bring it to my school. I felt that most people might find it too difficult. Some qi gong is a purely sitting meditation, for working on purifying your mind. Some qi gong works only on your body. And some qi gong works on both mind and body.

You should not need to separate these two exercises. Rather, think of both as brother and sister. I sometimes use qi gong as a warm-up before tai chi practice, and most students love it. I sometimes use tai chi movements while practicing qigong, so that my students can feel the *qi* (energy) in their bodies and hands. People who practice tai chi will sense the *qi* sooner when they practice qi gong as well; people who practice qi gong will learn tai chi more quickly and more easily.

For beginners, I suggest you practice qigong first; then start to learn tai chi after you feel the benefits of qi gong. This way, you will know that *qi* does exist and can be felt. But you should not feel restricted. You may start to practice tai chi anytime if you wish, as long as you understand that it is a long journey.

Both tai chi and qi gong can be used for healing the body and mind, to nurture the spirit, to strengthen internal energy, to boost the immune system, and to help you focus. Both of them can be your lifetime friends. Keep in mind the differences listed in the table below.

Differences between Tai Chi and Qigong

Tai Chi	Qigong
Advanced energy workout	Beginner energy workout
Needs full concentration to achieve full benefits	Needs full concentration to achieve full benefits
Movements are slow and circular, slow-paced with special form and specific steps. May initially be difficult to learn the sequence; it takes a long time to learn a complete routine or form; it takes even longer to master it.	Movements are simple and easy to follow, easy to learn, some forms can be repetitive. Foot placement is easy.

Movement only.	Some qigong involves self-massage.
Five main styles or forms: Yang, Chen, Wu', Wu, Sun, and some variations	Five categories but more than a hundred forms: Taoist, Buddhist, Confucian, Martial Art, and Therapeutic
Breathing is slow and deep, coordinated with each movement.	Breathing can be slow or fast. It varies in different forms of qigong.
Related to martial arts.	Related to natural medicine.
Mostly practiced in walking motion	Can be practiced in any position, mostly in a standing position
Not practical for severe illness.	Good for all kinds of illness, no restrictions.
Beginners may be easily frustrated.	Some people may find it too simple.
Strong and solid results, but may be deferred.	Immediate results; long-term practice provides better results.
It serves as a self-discipline.	It serves as a self-therapy.
Participants can be younger, but it is for all ages.	Participants; can be older, but it is for all ages and all ability levels

Please Note: The above is a loose comparison. It comes from my own experience but things are never really so black and white. The interpretation is not intended to be that rigid. You should experience each type of exercise for yourself in order to really understand the benefits of them. You might discover something different and more valuable in one or the other. Everything has multiple aspects. Some things are good for one person, and other things are good for different persons. Some exercises may be right for me, and other exercises may be right for you. My recommendation is that you try them for yourself and feel the differences. Try to find out what you enjoy about each of them. After you practice for a while, you may be surprised to discover something beneficial that other people may not have noticed.

4

The Way to Wise Living

Common Sense Practice

Common sense means "common knowledge we should know." But unfortunately, there are many people who don't have common sense anymore. Common sense may apply to some people, but not to everyone. Why is this?

We live in a dynamic world, and we often deal with dynamic people providing input of dynamic information. We all assume that we are smart and do things in a smart way. But we often lose our common sense to distraction, stress, illness or physical ailments, and emotional distress. Our focus is often on others—others' successes, others' problems, others' misleading information, and others we blame. We often forget to pay attention to ourselves. This causes us to lose common sense.

What is common sense? Common sense is listening and paying attention to ourselves and to our world. It is considering what is going on in our health and lives: what makes health fail; what makes life successful? It is knowing how to correct mistakes, how to make improvements, and how to assess our energy flow. *Am I balanced or imbalanced? What do I need to change to restore balance?* The bottom line is we need to know how to make energy flow better, our lives flow better, and our work flow better by paying attention to ourselves.

There are a thousand different ways to go to get to your goals. By following your common sense to choose the right way, you will get there sooner. I have people who ask me "How did you get to this point? What made you so smart?" I cannot say I am so smart. But I do follow my common sense; I observe, pay attention, catch myself when I falter; I am open even to things that are not in my field; I am willing to correct myself, willing to change. If one way doesn't work, I go another way. If one method doesn't work, I use another method. If a person makes me anxious, I choose to walk away and let him go his way. If a drug or herbs cannot help me, I use exercise and diet to help myself. If I realize my memory is getting worse, I do things to improve my memory … and so it goes. I have found that to go with the flow is better than to go against the flow in both my practice and my life.

Following common sense can help you in many aspects in life. It can help you relieve stress, do things more effectively, and find the right path.

A patient named Marianne came to see me for an initial visit. Just by looking at her, I said to myself, *What the heck did this girl go through?* She appeared so stressed; she looked older than her age; her hands were shaking; and her shoulders were up and tight. The first thing I said to her was, "Can you put your shoulders down?" She replied, "I didn't know my shoulders were up." She then dropped her shoulders and laughed at herself. I then asked her to relax and convinced her that nothing would go wrong here.

After collecting her information and examining her body's meridian pathways, I realized that most of her problems were from her worry, anxiety, and fear. These created blockages in the energy pathways in her body, causing poor circulation, inflammation, and degeneration. Her heart, kidneys, spleen, liver, and lung in meridian pathway all had blockages, and so did all the organs they were associated with, which is not always the case. She had arrhythmia; a bladder problem; a bowel problem; indigestion; anxiety; depression; low energy; and back, neck, and shoulder pain. She had so many problems that it was no surprise that she was depressed. To help her, I felt that I had a challenge.

Fortunately, I am not afraid of challenges; challenges make me learn more, gain more experience, convince me that anything is possible, and makes me strong. I do have many challenged patients. Some are challenged in their attitude, and some are challenged by their physical ailments. I did not limit Marianne's treatment to addressing physical problems and unblocking her energy merely to promote circulation in her body. I also spent time helping her relax her body and mind, educating her with Daoism, and teaching her simple qi gong exercise. I acted as a guide for her to find her own power and wisdom. Everyone has power, but not everyone knows it, and still others don't know how to use it. I merely opened a door for her and taught her to find her own power and how to use it. After six months, she was 90 percent better. A year later, she was a totally different person.

Another patient named Mark I worked with recently had an illness that was not getting better with treatment by his physician. He came to see me with many puzzle pieces. He was also very skeptical and very anxious. He was straightforward when he said, "Americans don't want to change. We don't believe anything else but 'go to doctors, use whatever doctors give us, whatever procedures they do to us, or accept whatever surgery they perform.' We like to do things fast—the quick fix—just get it done. We don't want to wait; we worry about everything—job, kids, retirement, security, career—we tense up if there is anything happening ..." Finally I had to say to him, "That is why you have heart disease."

In Chinese medicine, the heart is related to the mind and thought processes. If you have an overwhelmed mind, it affects your heart and heart energy. Some people might have heart disease; some people may have insomnia or anxiety. Some people may lose focus; some people may be forgetful, and some people may have poor circulation. I had to work with my patient not only to help his heart with Chinese medicine treatments, but also to educate him. I taught him techniques to balance his heart energy and to relax. This is a long journey, well worth traveling.

We always say, "Good things take time." Don't get discouraged if you fail several times as you try to put theory into practice. You will have many opportunities to get back on track and be successful. Even the most successful projects take time to progress from many failures to success. Time allows you to learn; time allows you to heal; time allows you to forgive others; time allows you to bring back common sense; and time allows you to find happiness. Time nourishes your spirit. We should not waste time, and should use it wisely because it is so valuable. Time is like a river. It flows only in one direction.

R. L. Wing's translation of the Dao (Tao Te Ching), *The Tao of Power: Lao Tzu's Classic Guide to Leadership, Influence, and Excellence* says,

The brain accepts all types of information from all stimuli simultaneously, and the mind processes it in the form of emotional responses, intuitive feelings, and logically formulated analyses. In the West, we rely almost exclusively on logical analysis. We are encouraged to think in a linear fashion, using words and numbers to draw conclusions about our work and our lives. These logical functions, according to neurological research, are performed by the left hemisphere of the brain. At the same time, we learn to discount aesthetic or intuitive information—a right hemisphere function—because it is considered less valuable to our culture. Thus we find ourselves primarily concerned with measuring events and analyzing their meaning, rather than creating and directing their flow. We are taught to ignore the intuitive or irrational, no matter how strong these "gut feelings" might be. As these right hemisphere feelings are repressed, we lose touch with our intuitive mind, and our insights become increasingly rare. (p. 15)

The Secrets to Happiness

Happiness helps our brains and bodies maintain balance, and it prevents brain and body aging. You can see a person aging fast if she is not happy. Everyone deserves happiness, but not everyone knows how to find it. It cannot be found from another place, another person, another job, or another planet. It is from you. *You make happiness happen.*

When a person is not happy, there are three things that may need to be addressed. The mind may be troubled, tangled, or disturbed by negativities that make your spirit low. The energy flow in your body may be blocked, stagnant, or not flowing properly. You may have lost direction toward your goal. You may have one, or two, or three of these. When a person is happy, the mind is clear and healthy. The body's energy is harmonized and flows smoothly.

1. Exercise regularly.

Many people try to eat well to restore their health. Many publications emphasize dieting and nutrition. Eating well is absolutely important, but it is not enough to focus on diet only. I have many patients who spend lots of money for supplements, but still do not feel well. Our bodies are made of many joints, muscles, organs, and tissues, and all these are available for moving! We have to move in order to stay healthy. In my experience, exercise is more important than diet alone.

There are both Western and Eastern forms of exercise you can choose. Jogging, walking, running, swimming, tennis, ball games, hiking, tai chi, qi gong, martial arts, aerobic exercises are all beneficial to our brains. The bottomline is, you have to move your body.

2. Keep a positive attitude.

Our brains have such power to control our lives. The brain controls the mind; the mind controls behavior; behavior is the vehicle that drives life in many different directions. Our brains and minds can make all the difference in life. They can make our lives miserable or make our lives brilliant. They can destroy us; they can destroy others. They can bring a lifetime of happiness and success. There is a Daoist story about different mind processes:

Three men were walking down the road. They were passing a corner and saw a spider climbing the wall. Because the wall in that area was wet, the little spider fell down. The little spider climbed up a second time, then fell again; it climbed and fell repeatedly. Watching the little spider made all three men think about their own lives.

The first man thought, "My life is like this little spider: climbing all my life and always falling."

The second man thought, "Look at that: life is full of mistakes. If we took a moment, we could find different ways to do things. This little spider could find another place to climb where the wall is dry; then it might reach the top of the wall."

The third man thought, "I am so affected by this little spider. It does not give up! Even after falling so many times, it continues to climb with seemingly unlimited energy. If I can do this, I am sure I can succeed."

The story tells us that different thoughts create different directions we can take in our lives. Here's another story from the Dao:

A man had traveled a long way, after preparing for a long time, to take a test to become a government officer. The night before the test, he had three dreams while staying in a hotel. The first dream was that he was planting vegetables on a high wall; the second dream was that he was holding an umbrella over his head while he wore a rain hat; the third dream was that he was asleep next to a woman he loved, but back to back. He realized these three dreams were strange and needed to be interpreted and found a man who clamed he could interpret the dreams.

The man said to the dreamer, "Your life is dull; you plant vegetables on a wall, you are wasting your energy; you wear a rain hat, but you also carry an umbrella, you are doing useless work. You have a lover, but you are back-to-back sleeping on the bed; how can you make love?"

This man who had prepared for the test was very upset, depressed and disappointed; he decided not to take the test. He gathered his luggage to go home. The hotel owner saw him packing then asked him, "Why are you leaving for home; aren't you supposed to take a test today?"

The man told the hotel owner about the three dreams and their interpretation. The hotel owner said to him, "I know how to interpret dreams too, and you had good dream. The first dream tells you that your position will be high; the second dream tells you that you are assured to have total coverage; the third dream tells you it is time to turn around."

The dreamer felt much more confident after he heard this explanation.

He decided to go forward and take the officer test. He did very well too, and passed it. A year later, he got a good gomenment job.

This story tells us that life is a test: you can move forward or you can quit, depending on your mindset and how you think about things.

We live in a world with negatives and positives. If we focus on the negatives, it makes us vulnerable, prohibits us from moving forward, blocks our energy channels, and makes us feel down, debilitating us and making us old. As soon as we change the focus, things change, life changes, work changes, the whole world changes.

Being positive is the way to success and happiness. If you have a positive attitude, and take positive action, you most likely will be successful in whatever you do. If you fail, you can always get up and start over again; failure can teach us what doesn't work. Failing is a part of life's journey; there is no such thing as "never failing."

When you have a positive attitude, people like to be with you. They feel cheerful, and they feel good when you are around. Not many people like to be with someone who is negative. You lose friends that way. When you have no friends, depression becomes more pronounced. It is like a negative circle; everything becomes worse and worse. Without a change in attitude, or a change in the way of thinking, even antidepressants are less likely to be helpful.

A former patient of mine had clinical depression. His main problem was too much negativity in his mind and mental processes. He could not see the positive side of things, and we know that everything has two sides. He lost friends one after the other, and he lost girlfriends one after the other. He continued to feel lonely and frustrated; he continued to feel powerless and hopeless. He had no energy, no job, complained about his illness all the time, and blamed his doctor for being unable to help him. He felt he was unable to work. He refused to do qi gong, tai chi, or any other exercise. He complained that medications gave him many side effects, but he wanted to continue to use them. He continued to sink into the darkness, feeling depressed even though he went to a therapist on a weekly basis. This kind of person is very difficult to treat, because he does not have a positive mental attitude and is not willing to change his way of thinking. He would not let go of the negativity in his life, and he would not get better.

3. Don't be afraid of hard work.

People have told me many times, "You work hard." Yes, I work very hard and learn very hard too. Living in two different countries with so many changes, there is so much to learn. Hard work can be a good learning experience, and the more you do, the more you learn. Some people complain that they work too hard. If you don't enjoy what you are doing, the complaint is reasonable. However, many studies tell us that over 90 percent of healthy older people worked hard in their lifetimes and volunteered in later life as well. If you enjoy the work you do, even if it is hard work, it can be still be rewarding. If you complain about everything you do, you are in trouble, and it is wise to seek help. Complaining creates negative energy that not only makes you unhappy, but affects other people as well. You should look for enjoyment in working with different people, being exposed to different knowledge, and getting paid for your hard work.

Working is part of learning. Even if you don't like what you do, you are still learning; even if you don't get paid well—or not paid at all—you are still learning. You may not realize the learning part at the moment, but you will realize it when you start dealing with things by yourself, because you will be smarter dealing with them.

4. Be honest with yourself, and with others.

Honesty is an important part of living in harmony. It would make the world different if we were all honest. Honesty creates trust; trust creates harmony; harmony leads to happiness. If people lose trust in family, friends, business associates, or politicians, it creates problems in our lives and in society. Losing trust is very negative. It does not bring good results.

Many of my patients have said to me, "I have trust in you; I know you can help me." This kind of mindset makes my work easier. It allows me to perform my best, and to make the healing work more effectively too. My father always told me, "Always be honest. You have nothing to lose." I grew up in an honest family. I studied medicine with an honest heart, and I do business in an honest manner. I treat patients with honesty. If I cannot help a patient, I tell the truth. This makes my life a lot easier and less stressful, and my patients appreciate being treated with respect.

Some people play mind games and try very hard to figure out what to say or what to do. They modify their behavior because they are afraid of being criticized. This creates blockages. They don't understand that if they are honest, they have nothing to fear. Constant tension creates stress and blockages in your energy system and also makes your life tiring and stressful. You cannot be truly happy when you carry tension and stress.

5. Help other people.

Human beings have a long history of helping each other in order to survive and live. For example, in China, families help each other, friends help each other, and co-workers help each other. Even in the past, when they had lower incomes, the Chinese were considered a "happy culture." Now, that culture of happiness continues in most rural areas and provinces.

In the United States, privacy seems most important in many people's lives. A while ago, my husband and I were walking in the woods. By accident, we walked into a neighbor's property. It was a huge wild place next to a public road. While I was contemplating the beautiful place, a man came out to tell me that the place we were walking belonged to him and asked us not to walk there anymore. I felt very humiliated in front of this young man. But I also felt bad for him, because I know that his kind of mindset cannot create a happy life. It doesn't matter how big a yard he has, how much money he has, or how rich he is, he will have many other issues. A happy person always has a heart for other people.

A friend of mine accidentally cut a dead tree in her neighbor's yard, and the neighbor filed a lawsuit for two thousand dollars against her. My question was, "Is a dead tree more important than friendship with a neighbor?"

From many years of observation and experience, I have found that people who tend to give more are happier than people who tend to take more. When you help other people, or give to people, you get a psychological reward from being able to give to others. The positive action makes you feel good and happy. If you think you lose something by helping others, or if you are worried that you are giving too much and not getting back, or if you try to calculate whether it is fair or not fair, you create tension and stress that causes blockages in your body, in your mind, in your life, in your relations, and in your health. The calculation of "how much do I get?" weakens your spirit. Give for the sake of giving, and don't feel the need to get back. Giving is priceless if it is from your heart, and nothing can measure the value. You will be a lot happier, because you will know you have something to offer. Life is about *creating* happiness, not getting it.

I sometimes do volunteer work for nonprofit organizations, even if I have to postpone my own work. Volunteering is not a waste of my time, because I enjoy working with other people and learning new things too. I enjoy being productive and generous for something I believe in, and I enjoy the group energy. This has had a very positive impact on my spirit, and I have learned a lot from all kinds of group activities.

6. *Avoid over analyzing.*

There are major differences between the Western mind process and the Daoist mind process. It is the same difference as the left-brainer practice and the right-brainer practice. This is not about which one is better; it is about wisely using the wisdom of both, because both Western and Eastern mind processes both have strengths.

The Western mind process tries to analyze everything, trying to figure out why and how we need to respond. But in some cases, when you try to analyze, or try to find the exact answer, you over-analyze and create an ongoing battle within yourself. You may understand the cause of the problems, but you may not know how to get rid of them. Things happen for many reasons and can be solved in many different ways.

Daoist mindset uses the Daoist philosophy to correct the imbalance in your mind, to help you to let go of whatever is bothering you, and thereby preserve your energy and your spirit. It is intuitive rather than logical. You follow your intuition and common sense, rather than over-analyzing. You live with flow; or as we often say, "Whatever floats your boat." There is wisdom there.

I had a patient named Jessica with many mental and emotional issues. She had been seeing a psychotherapist all her life and still had many problems. She was unable to let go of the negatives of the past. She totally understood where her problem came from, but she could not make things better. She still blamed her parents for causing damage to her life in her childhood. She held onto negative thoughts that caused worry and prohibited her from doing many positive activities. She worried about things that would probably never happen, which was a complete waste of energy. Caution is good to have in order to deal with situations that are unexpected. But worry creates negativity that takes energy away from you, creates blockages in your body's energy pathways, and debilitates you. We don't need extra worry that troubles our health; our minds are already too busy from too much information. People think too much, worry too much, plan too much, and fear too much. This behavior creates stress and tension and can trigger depression, anxiety, and panic attacks.

The Dao teaches us to relax, to let go of negatives, to find balance and inner peace, to discover the power inside of you, to find your wisdom and let it guide your way to light. You cannot control everything that happens, and you cannot predict everything that happens. The more you analyze, the more problems you may have. I suggest you try not to waste energy this way, but try to preserve energy for more important work, such as improving health, happiness, and well-being. When things happen, find ways to deal with them practically and in the moment. I recommend that you practice this way of thinking, and I am sure you will find things are definitely better.

7. *Forgive Others, Forgive Yourself*

> *True forgiveness includes total acceptance. And out of acceptance, wounds are healed and happiness is possible again.*
>
> —*Catherine Marshall*

Forgiving others can create positive energy and help you to heal, to let go, to move on, and to succeed. We all make some mistakes in our lives, and we all can learn from our mistakes. Love can create forgiveness, and forgiveness can nurture love.

> *Only the brave know how to forgive; it is the most refined and generous pitch of virtue that human nature can arrive at. A coward never forgives; it is not in his nature.*
>
> —*Laurence Sterne, Sermons*

Some people tend to hold onto insignificant and negative things. Letting go of unpleasant things that happened in your past can make your life easier. When you hold onto negative things, you lock yourself in a cage, and you have no freedom. Once you are able to let go, you set yourself free. Your energy channels are opened, your mind is free, and your happiness returns. Try to remember that every day is a new day, a new life. Life is like water constantly flowing with no end. It flows in one direction and does not flow back. We don't need to always bring the old things back, especially things that were not pleasant. When I talk about letting go of the old negative stories, some will argue with me: "We have to remember the history, so we can learn from history." Yes, we can learn from the history, but this should be in the context of a transformation from negative to positive, a change for the better. If we constantly remember the negative parts of history, it creates negative energy that misleads us and causes some degree of blockage in our emotions and mental processes; the learning is not going to happen. Remember, those unpleasant events are gone forever.

8. *Use Daoist wisdom in everyday life.*

I'll say it again: learning Daoist philosophy and living with Daoist wisdom can help you to become natural and spontaneous. You can then become more relaxed, accepting, tolerant, appreciative, and positive. Chinese people have used Daoism for centuries. In almost every field, people use Daoism to find the answers for their own needs. The military uses the Dao to make correct battle strategies. The scientist uses the Dao to figure out how to make things happen. Chinese doctors use the Dao to help patients get well in the most efficient way. Teachers use the Dao to provide quality and balanced teaching. Astronauts use Dao to stay focused and to follow scientific processes. Farmers use Daoism to predict the weather and follow the weather pattern to prepare for planting and harvesting. Chinese believe that if you use Daoist wisdom, your success rate is higher. We can take advantage of this philosophy and use this ancient wisdom to help ourselves. This wisdom does not directly tell you what to do, but it does give you a light and direction to help you see things more clearly. It teaches you to unload yourself, free your mind, and let things happen spontaneously and naturally. When you are really into Daoist practice, you are less likely to be affected by any kind negativity.

Here is a Daoist story about Zhuang Zi an influential 4th century Chinese philosopher :

> *A man asked Zhuang Zi, "You have been giving wisdom to others; your intelligence is superior—why is it you are not in a superior position?" Zhuang Zi replied, "The monkeys are playful in the big mountain; they can display their intelligence freely and nimbly. When they are in the jungle with so many thorns, they are helpless in moving their bodies, and unable to display their skills. But as soon as they go back to the mountain, they can display their skills again."*

The story tells us to accept the situation we are in and find the way that best suits our needs. It also tells us to be patient; each one has her own place to exhibit skill.

Generally speaking, the natural way cannot go wrong. If you are against the natural way, you may live with many "obstacles." In Daoist study and practice, you can be happy whether you are rich or poor, at any intellectual level or occupation, and at any age. In human healing, Daoist practice can accelerate healing. The bottom line is that you have to open your mind, open it to all possibilities, and don't hold onto things that are not helpful.

Again, from Wing's translation of the Tao Te Ching, *The Dao of Power*:

> *True power is the ability to influence and change the world while living a simple, intelligent, and experientially rich existence. Powerful individuals influence others with the force of example and attitude. Within groups, they have great presence—intellectual gravity—that*

influences the minds of those exposed to them. Intellectual gravity develops as a result of expanded identification—an identification that reaches far outside the self. Individuals who can identify with the evolution of reality develop significance and power because the force of their awareness is actively defining the universe around them. There are two major changes that occur in the lives of individuals who achieve personal power: the rise of intellectual independence and the need for simplicity. Daoism, as a way of understanding the universe, is not based on faith; it is based on experience. The human mind is evolving, while all social systems are temporary experiments. Relying on systems of understanding created or interpreted by others will dull the instincts and prevent individuals from cultivating and expanding their own minds.

9. Continue learning and keep your mind open.

We previously talked about learning. The more you learn the greater understanding you will have. I always tell people in my teaching, "The day you stop learning is the day you are deceased." Knowledge has more value than money—you can make money, but you must learn to gain knowledge. Knowledge can help you make more money. Giving a high priority to learning has been a tradition in China and Europe for many years. There are also many Americans who give learning priority. Since I was a child, I always liked to be around people who had vast knowledge or who just knew more than me. I felt like they were a source for me, teaching me to do things right and that things happen for a reason. I love to learn anything that can enrich my mind and help my understanding of the world.

When I was on a farm in China, I really admired the farmers who could predict the weather just by looking at the sky. I wanted to be like that. So I collected weather books, hand-copied information in my notebook, and started to look at the sky every day to try to predict the weather for the next day. Sometimes I got it right, but sometimes not. I was still an amateur. But the farmer got it right every time. I had fun being with knowledgeable people.

One obstacle to healing and happiness that many people have is a closed mind, especially to new things. People were taught in a certain way and continue that one way of thinking, generation after generation. Willingness to change goes together with a willingness to learn. As we discussed before, change is not a bad thing. In the past hundred years, the way we live has changed so much. Admittedly, some things changed for the better and some things for the worse, or at least became unpleasant, but eventually things always change to be good again. Everyone goes through changes as he matures. Some people are happier than others, and some people are more successful than others. Learning is an important part of making things change for the better. Open your mind, learn from many different sources, and learn from the past—but don't stay in the past! This will help you understand life better, see things from multiple angles, and make better decisions in all situations.

10. *Cherish love and friendship in your life.*

Love comes when we take the time to understand and care for another person.

—*Janette Oke.*

We all have the ability to give love and enjoy being loved. Love can be interpreted in ways other than just for husband and wife, boyfriend and girlfriend. Love between mother and daughter or son, love between friends, love between siblings, love between you and your pet, love between you and your parents are examples of the many possibilities. All love can be appreciated and cherished. There is an old saying in the Chinese culture: *Once you become a friend, you are a friend forever.* On one of my trips to China, a girl who has been my friend since middle school gave me a big punch as soon as she saw me. The reason she punched me was because I hadn't told her earlier that I was coming to China. I had to apologize ten times while laughing hysterically. Sometimes, people don't cherish friendships and may even abuse a friendship, which results in creating loneliness. Remember, if you give love, you also receive love. If you abuse friendships, you will never have true friends. Here is rule of thumb: *If you don't like other people to treat you unpleasantly and with disrespect, you should not treat them that way.*

I believe that sharing love, being honest with each other, forgiving each other, understanding each other, helping each other, taking care of each other, caring for each other, giving to each other, supporting each other, all help to avoid problems. Within a family, or if you live with one other person or several people, if you always think about *me, my comfort, my sleep, my pleasure, my life,* or *my needs,* without thinking much about other people's comfort, sleep, pleasure, life, or needs, then you will have unsuccessful relationships in marriage and friendship.

Love helps you understand better. With love, many problems can be solved.

We can do no great thing, only small things with great love.

—*Mother Teresa.*

5
Get with the Program, Stay Young

We have discussed so much about the whys and hows of health and happiness. Now, we need to put what we've learned into action. Without action, nothing can succeed; nothing will be done. Once a patient told me, "I still have your qigong DVD from five years ago, but I haven't tried it yet." So, what are the benefits of purchasing my qigong DVD? Another person said to me, "I love your book; I am going to follow your guidance in your book to help my weight." Then, I asked him, "When do you start?" He said, "I don't know yet." I preferred to hear him say "Next month," or even "Next year"; that would've been better than, "I don't know yet," which may mean never.

Many people are thinkers. They think and think, over and over, but nothing gets done. Some people are doers, and things do get done. Even if there is failure in doing it, they still learn to improve. I suggest that you do both. Think about your goal; make a plan for your goal. Then, make a plan of action for reaching your goal. When you finish, you will say to yourself, "I am glad I did that."

Learning Approach

There are two kinds of learning and practice: old school learning and new school learning. Old school learning emphasizes the practice of basics, and building a foundation before starting. In the Shaolin Temple's[5] early years, students had to carry water to the mountain every day for a certain number of days before learning any martial arts skill. In modern martial arts training, students need to do many kicks, punches, jumps, splits, and running, before learning any form of martial art. In learning tai chi, students need to do "cat walk", stance training, shifting, turning, and qigong practice every day for many days before learning the form.

New school learning focuses on form practice. Tai chi skill is actually built on practicing the form. When one form is learned well, other forms are easier to learn.

Both schools of learning have advantages and disadvantages. The old school learning is more difficult and boring and may lose students. But, this kind of learning definitely builds solid skills by building up a strong body and strong core energy. It is great for self-defense. The new school learning is a little easier, more flexible, and the focus on form makes it more fun. It is good for the brain and promotes new connections in brain cells. But the new school learning doesn't give you fighting ability. Since each individual has different needs, you can choose whichever way you want to learn.

Fundamental Principles of Tai Chi Practice

In order to have good study and practice, you need to understand tai chi's principles.

Once you understand the principles, learning becomes easier. Your tai chi journey will be easier, and you will develop better skills, have better health benefits, better *qi* circulation, and better martial skill. In the United States, there are more and more research studies being done on tai chi and qigong exercise, because of increasing awareness about tai chi and qi gong worldwide.

— Tai Chi Mental Status and Physical Postures

When you start tai chi practice, the first thing you need to learn is relaxation. It is easier said than done. In all the classes I have taught, I must have asked my students to relax a million times.

— Your Mind

Your mind comes first in learning, healing, and anti-aging. When practicing tai chi or qi gong, you need to *focus* on the body movements and energy

---

5   The Shaolin Temple, a monastery in Henan Province, China, is the home of the martial arts school of Kung Fu.

center. Don't let your *shen* (mind and spirit, in Chinese) walk away. You must focus solely on your own energy, and you will become determined. When you understand that *you* are on the way to your goal, you will do it without any hesitation.

Your mind's intention should be on tai chi or qi gong, with thoughts focused only on your body and relaxation. Once your mind is relaxed, your body becomes relaxed. If there is any tension, you need to get rid of it. Your eyes are not focused on any one object, but they take in full awareness of the surroundings. The mind produces *internal movement,* and internal movement produces *external movement.* All movements are directed from your mind. If your mind is not there, there will be no *qi.* Just as with anything else, if your mind is off track, you will not be able to do things successfully.

— Your Shoulders

Your shoulders should be relaxed. The elbows should be relaxed and about forty-five degrees from the body. If you elevate your elbows or shoulders, you create tension in your arms and shoulder area. From a martial arts standpoint, relaxing your shoulders and dropping the elbows is a protective strategy. If your shoulders are raised, your elbows will also be lifted. Then you are giving the opponent the chance to get you down or lock you up. Only if you are relaxed are you able to respond quickly to any movement by your opponent. Your arms should follow your body in every movement of tai chi. You do not intentionally move the arms; rather you let the arms go wherever the body goes. If you focus too much on your arm work, you look like you are dancing, rather than doing tai chi.

— Your Wrists

Your wrist should be relaxed and flexible, but well-controlled. Relaxed doesn't mean floppy and having no strength, and controlled doesn't mean rigid. This will give you more readiness to change any way you need to in a fighting situation. Although practicing tai chi is not designed for fighting, if you know it, you will have a self-defense tool to use in an urgent situation. Your hands should be relaxed with fingers slightly closed together.

— Your Torso, Back, and Legs

Your torso and back should be relaxed. If you can relax the back, it allows for a smooth flow of energy. Your back carries the important nerve system that directs all parts of your body. Keeping the back healthy is an important aspect in the prevention of health problems. If you are tense, you will create stagnation on the back meridians and the nerve system that is related to your whole organ system and body parts. No matter how you move your body, your back should be upright and relaxed. You will be very uncomfortable if your body is twisted or bent. You can get hurt or injured if you practice with an incorrect body posture. You can tuck the buttocks inward to keep the lower back straight.

From a martial arts point of view, the waist, or abdomen, is your *powerhouse*. When your abdomen is loose, the power generated by your legs can be easily transmitted to your arms through your waist. Your waist can also generate power that directly moves energy to your hands. If your waist is stiff or tight, the power generated from your legs cannot be transmitted to your hands. Your *"powerhouse"* therefore has less power. Ancient tai chi masters stated, *The root is at your feet, power is initiated by your legs and directed by your abdomen, then expressed through your hands.*

Your knees should be bent during the entire tai chi practice. You don't have to bend very low, however. For beginners or seniors, you can just unlock your knees. For advanced or younger people with a flexible body and strong legs, you can bend the knees a little lower. It depends on the individual's ability. Doing it correctly is more important than maintaining a low stance. With each shifting of weight and turning of the waist, you can clearly distinguish between substantial (full) and insubstantial (empty) yin and yang movement. Once you begin to understand the idea of substantial and insubstantial, you will have a centered and a balanced feeling, and be solid and grounded no matter what the movements may be. If you do not feel balanced, that means you just need to practice more.

Once you have relaxed all parts of the body, your entire body should be rooted, balanced, and centered, just like a tree. The strong roots of a tree can defend against a heavy wind or storm. Once the entire body relaxes, you will feel your internal "generator" is in standby mode, ready to generate the energy. This is a very important skill to learn in tai chi practice. It also helps you relieve stress, detach from all the junk in your mind, and let go of all tensions.

Tai chi is an entire body exercise and involves coordination of all body parts. Through tai chi practice, you will improve your coordination too. One tai chi principle from an ancient master states, *When there is an upward movement, then there is also a downward movement; when there is a left movement, then there is also a right movement.* Your body moves before your arm, your leg moves before your body. Each part of the body follows, one after the other.

— Your Breath

Breathing is important in both tai chi and qigong practice. Breathing should be deep and slow, and coordinated with the movements. In tai chi practice, the breath should be fully addressed in advanced students, but not in beginners, because it can cause confusion due to the complicated tai chi movements. As you practice for a while and master the whole form, you can start to pay more attention to your breathing. Generally speaking, you breathe out when you direct energy out; you breathe in when you bring energy in. Certain movements have different breath patterns, which you will learn eventually. Some breathing techniques in qigong can be confusing, especially if you have never learned *how to breathe correctly* before; but you will learn from your instructor. You should not be afraid to ask your instructor about breathing, any other difficult movement, or any other questions at all.

Tai Chi Basic Movement Requirements

Tai chi is a whole body exercise. Whenever there is movement, the whole body moves. When one part of your body moves, all other parts also move. There is motion in stillness, and there is stillness in motion in every movement. All movements are rooted in the feet, initiated from the leg, controlled by the waist, and shaped by the hands and fingers. Being rooted in your feet creates the strong roots of the tree, and then your legs start to move, followed by the waist. This is how it appears in movement.

The upper and lower parts of the body are coordinated; left and right are coordinated; mind and body are coordinated; breathing and movements are coordinated. Do not worry if you have poor coordination. It will improve with practice. All movements are in a circular and continuous motion. There are many things in the natural and physical world that are created and move in the shape of a circle, such as the earth, the moon, the sun, a cup, a dish, a ball, a wheel, your eye, most fruits and certain vegetables, pots and pans, and so many others. Many of them have energy. This is part of the reason why the circular motion is so important.

Your weight is continually shifting from left to right, and then from right to left. The waist position is also constant and continues turning from side to side. This describes the yin and yang of tai chi movements.

Tai Chi Practice Requirements
— Discipline

Developing tai chi discipline is very important in tai chi practice. It takes effort and mind power. You have to constantly remind yourself that you are a special person, your hard work will pay off, and you are not wasting your time. Discipline can take you to the place you want to be and can lead you to your goal.

— Patience

Nothing worthwhile comes easily overnight. Being frustrated only gets you down and make you sick. Tai chi learning is like a natural healing journey; it takes time. There is no short cut or quick way to learn. If you don't get it right this week, maybe you will next week, or next month, or next year. It doesn't matter how long it takes. Many people think that learning "the form" is all there is to tai chi study. To learn tai chi form is not the whole story. To learn it correctly may be difficult, and it may take a long time. But if you want to see the beauty of a mountain view, you have to plan a trip and hike to the top. This can be hard work, but then you will see the view. Many tai chi masters in China have studied for a lifetime and still practice regularly.

In Chinese martial arts, there is no belt awarded. The reward is inside the practitioner. When it's time for a real battle or tournament, you see the true and real skills. People look for shortcuts to success, but they really need to understand that shortcuts don't give you stability, or foundation. Only hard work and a solid foundation will bring true quality, real skill, and true benefits.

— Confidence

I have often seen the effects of lack of confidence. Confidence and pride are two different things. People who have too much pride may not have enough confidence. Confidence is within you. All you need to do is to use it. You cannot say you don't have it; maybe you just haven't found it. If you have a weakness in your confidence, it can be strengthened. Confidence comes from your mind and the way you think. Worry, fear, and laziness can diminish your confidence.

You can do anything if you put your mind to it. Everyone has strengths and weaknesses; there is no such thing as perfect. "Imperfection" is just another word for uniqueness. Everyone has had a different experience. Some people learn one thing quicker, and some people learn other things quicker. However, everyone can learn if they choose to learn, if they are determined to learn, and if they put their minds into learning. Just like when you go to college, you will graduate if you choose to graduate; you will get A's if you choose to get A's; and you will drop out if you choose to drop out. Healing and learning are the same. You might feel discouraged in the beginning, but once you practice for a while, your confidence will build up, and it will be stronger every year. The longer you practice, the more confidence you will have.

— Diligent Practice

Without diligent practice, you will not develop your tai chi skill, and you will not reach your goal. Compare a doctor, who just graduated from medical school and a doctor who has practiced for twenty years. Who would you choose? This is just a simple example. If you need a service from a company, would you choose a new company or a well-known company that has been providing the service many years? Remember, good skill comes from diligent practice. The practice of tai chi or qigong should be fun, and not a chore. If you think it is fun, you will practice regularly; doing it with others makes diligent practice a party.

— Non-Competitive

There is no competition in tai chi practice. There is no need for you to compare your skill to other people's skills. Tai chi is for health maintenance, disease prevention, the healing of illness, as well as for building inner peace and delaying aging. Don't worry if you see someone else's coordination is better than yours. So what? Watch and learn. You only compete with yourself to improve day-to-day, not with other people. There are no belts in tai chi practice. The real belt is measured by how you have improved over a period of time—in relaxation, coordination, physical health, emotional happiness, mental alertness, creativity, learning ability, relationships with others, and stability in your life style.

— Always Warm Up Before and Cool Down After

It is important to do warm-up exercises before practice and to cool down after practice. Especially, do the warm-up exercises described in this book, because they are designed specifically to stimulate your brain. You may choose any of the warm-up exercises you wish. I designed a series of warm-up exercises to help your qi and blood flow in your whole body and to loosen your muscles and joints. They also help to balance your emotions, enhance your brain-cell communication, and promote organ harmony. You can also use power-walking or jogging for a warm-up. It depends on each individual's needs, or on the convenience of the exercise. The warm up exercises speed heart rate and promote circulation which is another benefit to brain and prevent brain aging.

After practice, you should not immediately become inactive. You should let the muscles slowly cool down with the cool-down exercises in this book. If the muscles are warm, then suddenly become cool for a long period of time, it causes stagnation of the blood circulation and muscle stiffness, and it increases the possibility of muscle and tendon problems in the future. Some athletes have muscle stiffness and inflammation of the soft tissue due to improper cool-down.

— Frequent Practice

People often say, "I don't have time to do this." It is not about whether you have time or not. You might *never* have time. It is about whether you *make* time or not. It is about choosing a priority. If your priority is health, you choose to do things to be healthy, make time for health-related activities. If your priority is learning, you choose to learn, you make time to learn. If your priority is taking care of your family, you choose to do so. No matter what you choose, you may not be able to do it if you lose your health.

In preventive medicine, we encourage people to put a priority on health. When you lose your health, you lose everything. To truly get benefits from tai chi and qi gong, it is best if you can practice every day, even if it's just warm-up exercises or some movements from the warm-up exercises. At the very least, set your intention to practice three to five times a week. You don't need to feel bad if you miss practice once or twice. As long as you have the intention, you can make up for it at your next practice. You may find that your body misses practice; that is a good sign. You will know that you are doing something right for yourself. We call this a *healthy craving*. If you have a specific need, these exercises will meet your need. For instance, if you feel down, practice the Exercise for Emotion Balance, described in chapter six.

— Outdoor Practice

When practicing outdoors, avoid strong winds and extreme cold or hot temperatures. Strong wind and extreme cold distract your attention and affect energy flow around your body. It is difficult to get good circulation from tai chi practice in cold weather. If it is too hot, it might cause dehydration or heat stroke.

You should avoid wearing a hat during your practice. When you are bending forward, or practicing in a breeze, your hat may fall off your head, and to pick it up is a distraction. There is an acupuncture point on the top of your head called the Bai Hui point or Hundred Convergences point, on the governing vessel meridian. It receives energy from above, and then connects to all other energy channels in the body. You want that point open as you practice these qi exercises.

— Practice with a Group

As we discussed before, working with a group can generate better results. It is more fun too. Attending regular classes helps you learn good habits and correct routines. The positive social environment gives you positive feedback and reinforcement. If you cannot find a quality teacher, you can always start your own group. Following a videotape or DVD to learn is adequate, but more difficult. For learning tai chi, I designed a sequence called "Tai Chi Basics," which is great for beginners. It is the bridge to self-study of tai chi in any form. Self-study of qi gong is not difficult, as you can do it just by following a DVD. But, it is so much better if you can find a good instructor.

— Opposite-Side Practice

If you already know a tai chi form, and know it very well, you can start to practice opposite side, or "mirror side." It definitely enhances the connection of brain cells. It may feel very difficult in the beginning, but soon it will be great. You will then realize your overall ability is improving, as well as your memory. If you want to focus on the martial arts aspect of tai chi, it is ideal for you to do opposite-side practice to further stimulate both sides of your brain. You will get optimal benefits from this approach. If you are a beginner, this is a perfect way for you to exercise both sides of the brain. Don't worry how well you do. It only matters that you do it. Tai chi practice has no judgment; you do it at your own pace, and ability. You will benefit as long as you follow the guidelines and principles.

There is other important information that can be learned from my book, *Natural Healing with Qigong*.

6
Four-Step Practice

Before you start to practice, check yourself for tension, weakness, and energy level. Where do you have fear or worries, and what is your relaxation level or stress level? Then, start your warm-up exercise. You do not have to do all of the movements described in this book; feel free to choose only some of them, but no harm will be done if you do them all. Then, choose some qigong movements. Again, you don't have to do all of them. It depends on your time availability. Doing just these exercises will give you plenty of benefit, so it is fine to not go any further at the beginning of your practice. But at some point, it is important to begin to practice tai chi.

After you practice, check yourself again for tension, weakness, and energy level. Do you still have fear or worries; what is your relaxation level now? Have these improved? Developing your awareness of these things will encourage and empower you to master your health and life. This awareness will anchor you to new learning and harmonize your brain multi-dimensionally, especially activating the frontal lobe.

The four steps for practice are Warm Up Exercise, Qigong Exercise, Tai Chi Practice, and Cooling Down Relaxation.[6]

---

6   The description of these movements with accompanying pictures can be purchased separately. Please visit www.ChineseMedicineforHealth.com to find out more or call (508) 429–3895 to purchase "True Brain Fitnes II, Practice Workbook".

Step One: Total Body Warm-Up Exercises

I discussed earlier that warm-up exercise is very important. Especially, do the warm-up exercises described in this book. It is designed for multiple health benefits and healing. You can also choose other kinds of warm-up exercise if you wish, such as power walking, and jogging. It depends on individual needs, conditions, and availabilities.

I designed a series of warm-up exercises to help your *qi* and blood flow through your whole body, loosen your muscles and joints, help your emotions, enhance your brain-cell communication, activate cross-activity between left brain and right brain, and promote organ harmony. This sequence of warm-up exercises involves whole-body movements. You can go through all the movements or just some of them, depending on your availability of time and physical ability, or other needs. If you have trouble with certain movements, you can start out gently in the beginning and then gradually increase the intensity.

The warm-up can be done in fifteen o twenty minutes each time. If you have more problems in one area than another, you can spend more time there and focus on that area.

Total Body, 27 Movements Exercise

The total body, twenty-seven-movements workout described below is designed for energy, blood circulation, balanced emotion, and brain stimulation. It should be practiced before tai chi or qigong exercise. For more details, the full description and pictures of the movements are in a different book, which you can purchase through our office at (508) 429–3895 or visit our website at: www.ChineseMedicineforHealth.com.

1. Rock feet forward and backward.

Feet are shoulder-width apart and whole body is relaxed. Gently shift weight from heel to ball, then from ball to heel, for about a minute or two.

2. Rock feet forward and backward, lifting heels (you can raise hands too).

Same motion as above, just lift heel higher. One to two minutes.

3. Alternate swinging arms forward and backward.

Legs straight with right leg in the front of left; swing arms forward and backward alternately as you shift weight from front to back of the leg.

4. *Rotate shoulders, while shifting weight.*

Maximum rotation of both shoulders backward four times; then forward four times. As you are rotating shoulders, your chest moves too. This is done while shifting your weight from one leg to the other.

5. *Circle arms back and forth (while shifting weight).*

With feet shoulder-width apart, and nothing within an arm's length on any side of you, shift weight from side to side. At a moderate to fast pace, circle whole arms alternately backward eight times; then circle arms forward eight times; repeat above movement several times in big circles like learning to swim.

6. *"Wax on, wax off" (vertical, horizontal arms).*

With palms facing front, in flexed position, alternately circle arms in the front of body, like wiping off dirt from a wall. Horizontally circle arms alternately with palm facing down, like wiping a table.

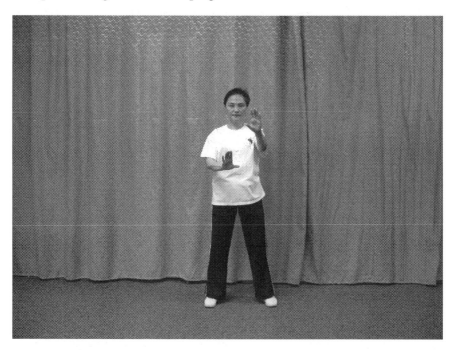

7. Simple arm pressing.

Use your right forearm to press on your left upper arm in the front of the body for 30 seconds; then use your left forearm to press on your right upper arm in the front of the body for 30 seconds

8. Pressing arms, move upper body.

This movement is not easy to do; you may feel awkward. Press arms as in the above movement, then move the body in a circle; reverse the circle after four times. Move the body in a horizontal figure-8. You feel like you are drawing (with your hand) a circle, and a horizontal number 8.

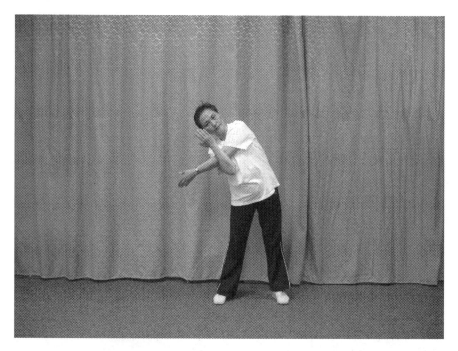

9. Wrists rotation.

This is not a difficult movement. Just rotate your wrist one after the other. You can move your body at the same time if you so desire. Do it free-style with footwork—like a disco dance!

10. *Tendon stretching.*

A. Lift both hands and left leg, then step down slightly in front of you as you bring your hands down by your sides, lean slowly forward to stretch right Achilles tendon. Lift hands and left leg again, then put left foot straight down next to right foot and bend both knees as if getting ready to jump. Do the same thing on other side with right leg up and lunge, stretching left Achilles.

B. Lift hands and left leg and then step to left as you bring your hands down by your sides; stretching both Achilles' tendons. Lift hands and left leg again and then bring you left foot down right next to your right foot and bend at the knees. Do the same thing on other side.

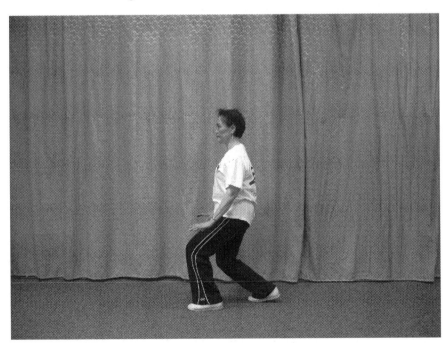

11. X-lifting:

Lift right elbow and left foot; put left foot down as both forearms cross in front of lower abdomen.

Lifting left elbow and right foot; put right foot down as both forearms cross in the front of lower abdomen.

Repeat several times.

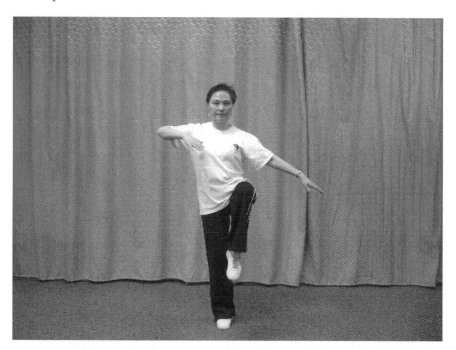

12. Reach sky, touch earth.

With feet together, reach high with both hands, while rising onto tiptoes; then with feet flat on the ground and bent knees, bend slowly over and place both hands on the floor. You neither have to touch the floor nor rise onto toes, if you are unable.

13. Funnel circle.

Feet together, standing straight with good posture. Hands together above head, with an imaginary string attached between them, you feel that your body is lifted. Circle hands while you keep your body still, like making an imaginary funnel over your head.

14. Hip rotation.

Bend both legs slightly. Rotate hips clockwise four times; then counter-clockwise four times. Just like using a Hula-hoop, but not as fast.

15. Touch opposite leg and foot

Touch opposite leg and foot alternately. You might have done this movement in an aerobics class or in a Brain Gym session. Right hand touches raised left leg. Then left hand touches raised right leg. Then repeat touching foot this time.

16. X-walk forward and backward.

Walk forward with left foot crossing the right foot, and right foot crossing the left foot four times, like a model walking down a runway. Walk *backward* with left foot crossing behind the right foot and right foot crossing behind the left foot. But be careful of what's behind you!

17. X-jump forward and backward.

Same theory and movement as above, but jumping, instead of walking. This requires some coordination and no obstacles underfoot. Take precautions!

18. Jumping, crossing hands and feet.

Jump up once and bring feet slightly apart and arms straight out to sides (open position) at shoulder level; jump again crossing feet with left foot in the front of right while crossing hands in the front of lower abdomen. Then repeat, with right foot crossing in front.

Then jump with feet wide apart again, arms open at shoulder level; and jump again crossing feet with right foot in the front of left, while you cross hands in the front of lower abdomen. Repeat on other side.

Repeat sequence five to ten . times or more.

19. Jumping, crossing hands high and feet opposite.

This is a similar movement to the above, except now hands and feet cross at opposite times. This is kind of fun as it takes time to get the hang of it. Jump up with feet apart, while *crossing arms overhead*; jump again and cross feet, left foot in the front of right, with arms open at shoulder level.

Jump again feet wide apart, now with hands crossed over the lower abdomen. Jump again and cross feet with right foot in the front of left, and arms open at shoulder level Repeat above five to ten times.

20. *Knocking method massage.*

Cross both hands, knock gently on opposite sides of the body: upper arm, forearm, wrist, head, shoulder, hip, and leg, waking them up.

21. *Airplane.*

It sounds a little exotic, but it is easy to do. Place arms out at shoulder level. Move the body in circle while keeping arms still.

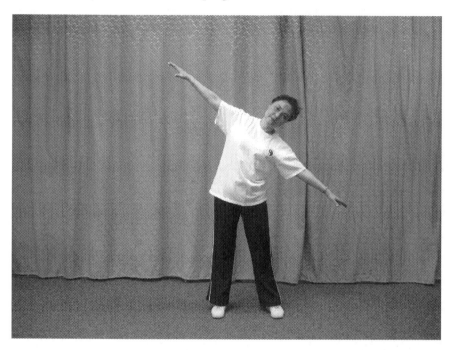

22. *Buddha holding qi:*

Stand in horse stance, with feet wide apart, knees bent, and pelvis tucked under. Put hands palms up on side of the body below shoulder level and relax whole body; focus on deep and slow breathing.

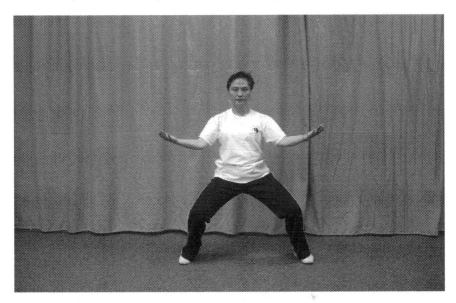

23. *Side lunge, alternately shifting weight.*

Start in horse stance—feet wide apart, knees bent, and pelvis tucked under. Slowly shift weight to left, then to right. Continue shifting weight from side to side. Stay on each side for 30 seconds.

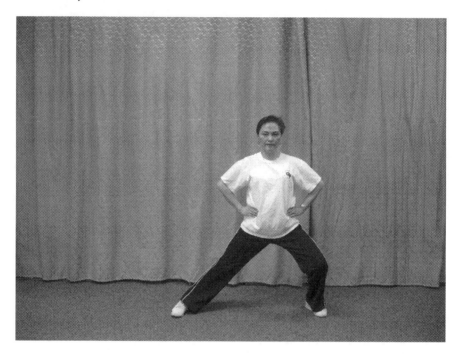

24. *Upside-down Y with deep breathing.*

Open feet wide, two times shoulder width, with legs straight. Interlock fingers above head with arms straight. Focus on deep breathing. Step forward with right leg in front, keeping arms overhead; focus on deep breathing, letting the breath go through your body. Bring right foot back and step left foot forward, while maintaining your arms overhead and your focus on the breath.

25. *Lunge and bending forward:*

Step with your with left into a forward lunge. Take a deep breath, raise hands above your head, breathe out, and move your hands down to the floor, keeping both knees straight if you can. Repeat four times.

Lunge forward with right foot in the front. Inhale, raise hands above head, breathe out, and move hands down to floor, keeping both knees straight if you can. Repeat four times.

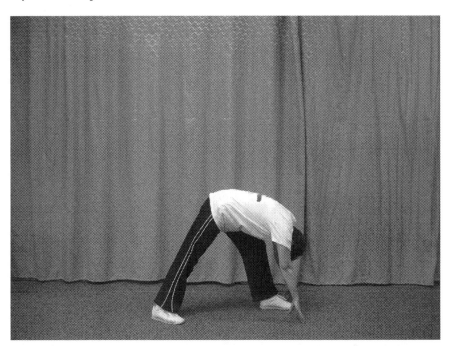

26. Chinese "Big," deep breathing.

If you know the Chinese character for *big* [大], you'll have no problem doing this movement. Place feet apart at two times shoulder width; place arms out at shoulder level and breathe through the body. With your palms facing down, imagine drawing energy up from the earth as you breathe. With palms facing up, imagine them filling with energy from the sun and universe.

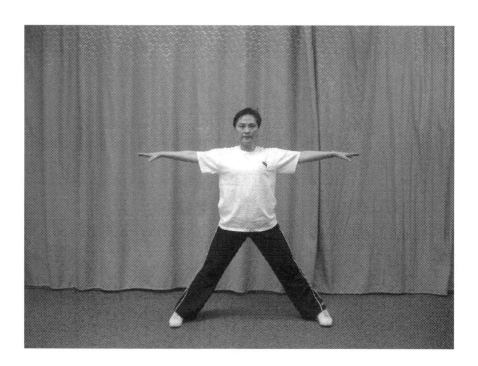

27. Shaking hands and feet, ending.

Shake hands vigorously; then shake one leg and then the other; shake arms and body vigorously, about one minute. Take three deep breaths, you have finished the total body warm-up practice!

Step Two: Qigong Practice for Special Purposes
— Qigong Exercise for Brain and Memory

This exercise group helps to balance both sides of the brain, the upper and lower parts of the brain, as well the midbrain. These exercises, when performed in conjunction with tai chi practice, enhance brain efficiency and memory. When I do these exercises regularly, I can really feel the difference in my mind process, my emotions, and my memory.

1. *Move qi through your body.*

Feet are shoulder-width apart. Raise arms up from sides of the body, and then bring arms down in front of the body. Imagine, as you are doing this movement, that you are gathering universal energy and allowing it to go through your body. Repeat three to five times.

2. *Push up, open the sky.*

Inhale and raise arms up in front of the body as if you are pushing up a weight. Visualize that you are lifting the energy from the earth and letting it move through your body, to your head, and then connecting that energy with the heavens.

Exhale and open arms to the sides while lowering them, opening to the energy of the universe. Repeat five times.

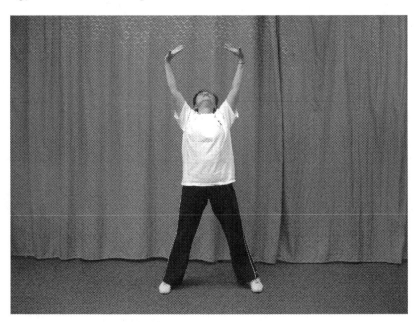

3. Shift body weight side to side.

Stand with good posture, feet shoulder-width apart and shift your weight to one side and then the other. As you do this, you can either wave your arms above your head, gently roll your neck, or lift and drop your shoulders, whichever feels right for you.

This practice helps to balance yin and yang. In Brain Gym theory, body side-to-side is one of the checks for noticing *laterality dimension,* which means the effective communication between the left and right hemispheres (including the frontal lobe and the sensory motor cortexes) as well as the left and right sides of the body.

4. Horizontal 8 moving the ball.

This is a tai chi skill practice for left and right brain hemispheres. Put one hand above the other, like holding a basketball. Turn your body toward upperhand; than exchange hands while turn body to opposite side. It looks like you are moving the ball in a horizontal figure-8,

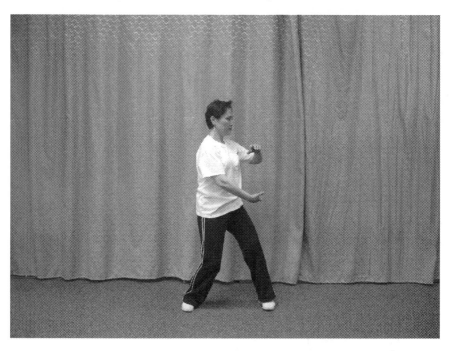

5. *Touch sky, touch earth.*

Inhale while you reach high with both hands; then touch the floor as you exhale. This movement is checking your *center dimensionality,* as well as working to stimulate the midbrain. It helps to move qi through the body more efficiently. When you touch the floor, you stretch your Achilles' tendon while your natural posture performs massage on your internal organs.

6. *Front back, rock feet.*

We mentioned this movement previously. This is a good balance practice. This gentle movement is checking focus dimension, working with brain stem, and cerebellum. You can either just rock back and forth, or rising onto toes and heels while you are rocking.

7. *Standing X Pose.*

Stand with feet two times shoulder width, raise your arms above your head and open wide, so your whole body makes the letter X. Inhale and exhale deeply five times. X-pose is an excellent qi practice, as well as a brain exercise. It allows all your channels to open, so your body can receive energy from the universe through them.

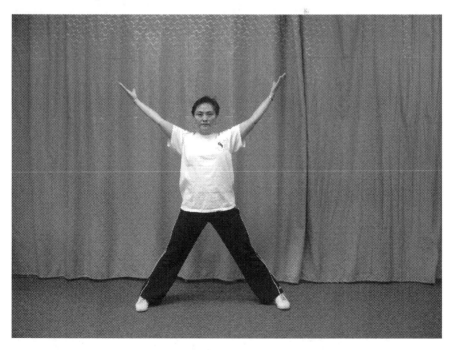

8. Folding X.

Once know how to do standing X pose, you will have no problem doing the folding X. Just bend your body forward and put your hands on your feet.

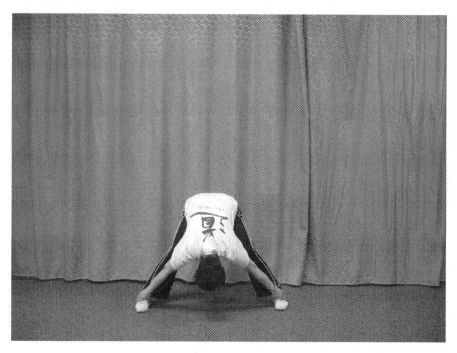

9. Two-dimension twisted X pose.

It is same pose, but you place your feet in front and back. This is also an excellent brain exercise, working on space orientation.

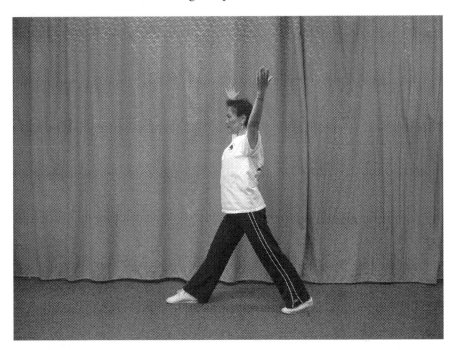

10. Folding two-dimension X pose:

While you're in the above pose, slowly bend forward until you touch the floor. If you have to bend your front knee when you touch the floor, that's okay. This is also an excellent brain workout for improved space orientation.

11. Circle knees in two directions.

This coordination legwork takes a lot of practice to master. This is not only an excellent brain workout because it involves multiple brain tasks, but also an excellent joint exercise. Don't you love things with multiple benefits? Circle one knee inward direction while you are circling the other knee outward direction.

12. Head massage.

There are many meridians and points that go though the head; these meridians are related to the brain and brain chemicals. By stimulating them with massage, you send signals to the brain and brain cells, increasing brain communication. Massage your forehead and temple area, the top, back and base of the scalp, and then your whole head.

13. Neck movement with eyes following.

Slowly turn your head to the left, to the right, up, and down, with your eyes always following in the direction of each movement. Repeat eight times.

14. In-motion hook-up.

This movement has multiple benefits: brain exercise, qi exercise, coordination exercise, stretching, and more. Cross feet and hands; interlock fingers; then turn wrist inward then upward until fingers point up. Take a deep breath; exhale bending forward and while reversing above movement: moving hands inward, then downward until fingers face down. Inhale and raise body and arms until your hands are above your head, with fingers still interlocked. Exhale, bending forward and moving arms down. Inhale; rotate interlocked hands inward. Exhale and bring body upright with interlocked fingers up and in front. Drop hands, uncross feet, and relax shoulders and whole body. Repeat this motion for four times.

— Qigong Exercise for Emotional Balance

This group of qigong movements helps to relieve anxiety, depression, high stress caused by emotional imbalance, and panic attacks. Some of these movements have been explained previously.

1. Turn body from side to side.

Feet are set shoulder-width apart, stand straight with arms and neck relaxed. Turn your upper body from side to side, allowing your arms to swing freely. Repeat this as many times as you feel like.

2. Release liver energy.

In a horse stance position—feet wide apart, knees bent, and pelvis tucked under—inhale and put both fists at waist level. Exhale and quickly, but without jerking your shoulder, move your *right fist* forward, just like you are punching a ball in front of you; then place your right fist back at your waist, inhaling. Exhale and quickly move your *left fist* forward like you are punching a ball in the front of you. Repeat this as many times as you want.

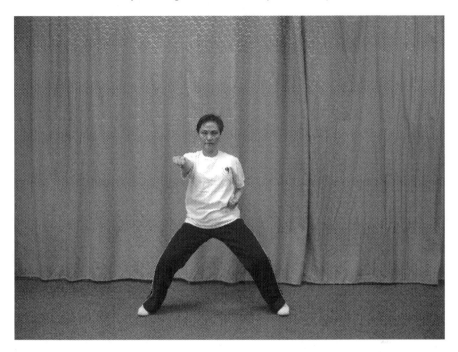

3. Standing X Pose (open all channels).

As we discussed before, X pose is an excellent qi practice, as well as brain exercise. Because this pose allows all channels to open, your body receives energy from the universe through the channels, as you focus on deep breathing. Opening your energy channels helps to remove the stagnation that causes emotional problems.

4. Chinese "big," palms up.

We discussed this pose before. Stand with your feet apart and your arms open wide at shoulder height. Focus your mind on your up-facing palms, imagining you are receiving energy from the universe. You will feel warmth in your palms.

5. Chinese "big" palms down.

Focus your mind on your down-facing palms, imagining you are drawing energy from the earth. You will feel warmth in your palms.

6. Connect upper and lower Dan Tian.

There are several *Dan Tian* in the body, all very important focal points for your center of gravity and your overall energy health. This position concerns the ones at your heart center and below your navel. Put your right hand on your sternum (in the center of your chest just above your solar plexus) and your left hand on your lower abdomen. Focus your mind on the connection between these two energy centers while breathing in and breathing out for a minute or two.

7. Cross hands and feet.

Cross your wrists and interlock your fingers. Put one foot across the front of the other. Take a deep breath while you turn your wrists inward; breathe out and continue to rotate your wrists until your elbows point downward and your hands point up. Relax your shoulders, elbows, and wrists. Keep fingers interlocked and hold, breathing in and out for a minute or two.

8. *Grab hand behind head, bend sideways.*

Take a deep breath and use your right hand to grab your left wrist behind your head; now breathe out and lean your body to the right. After two breaths, relax your body and arms.

Take a deep breath and use your left hand to grab your right wrist behind your head; now breathe out and lean your body to the left. After two breaths, relax your body and arms. Repeat two or three times on both sides.

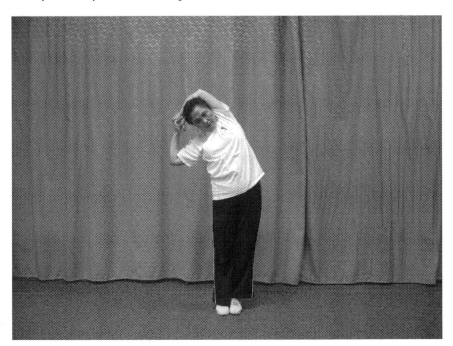

9. *Y blossom.*

This requires your mind to be present.

Put your feet together, and your arms up and open like a funnel shape. Your feet are rooted and receiving energy from the earth. Your arms are straight and relaxed, allowing the energy of the heavens to go down through your fingers, palms, and arms, move through your body, and then connect to the energy from the earth.

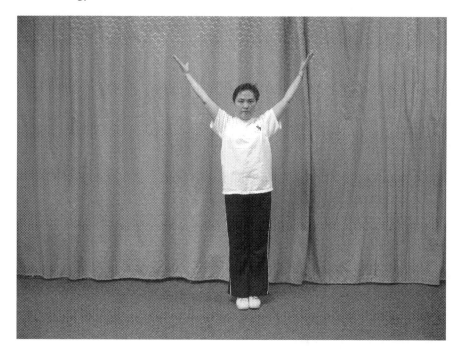

10. Acupressure liver point.

Put your palms at the side of your chest with thumbs on the front of ribcage and fingers at the back. With your thumbs, find the point that feels sensitive and press on it. Gently move your arms back and forth several times. Or you can just put pressure on these points.

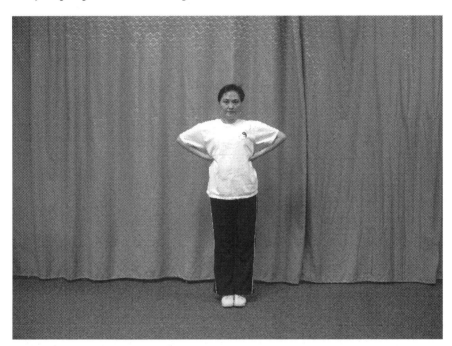

11. Arm massage.

There are six meridians that go through the arms, three meridians on each side with many energy points. These meridians connect to your organs. When you massage the arms, you are actually stimulating these meridians and points. Use one hand to massage the opposite arm, making sure to massage the whole arm. Change hands and arms after several minutes.

12. Ear massage.

You ears are like a miniature body. They have many points, which correspond to various body parts. Massage your ear, and you are indirectly massaging your whole body.

Step Three: Tai Chi Practice

— Tai Chi Foundation Practice: Tai Chi Basics, Tai Chi Qigong

Both tai chi basics and tai chi qigong are designed to help beginning students to build a tai chi foundation. As you practice, it will be easier. If you need more help, DVDs with further instruction are also available from our clinic.

— Tai Chi Basics:

If you practice tai chi basics for a while, you will learn the tai chi form easily. This will build a foundation for tai chi practice. Students show a big difference with and without tai chi basics, almost an amazing difference. I strongly recommend that you start with tai chi basics if you are just beginning. These exercises build on each other in sequence.

1. Shifting weight.

This is an easy movement. Set feet shoulder-width apart. Slightly unlock knees, put your weight on the left side, and then shift to the right side. Continue shifting weight from left to right, right to left for one or two minutes.

2. Shifting and turning.

This is based on the above movement, and adds turning the body to add more dimensions to the movement. You shift weight first, and then turn body to same side. Then to the other side, and so on.

3. Right hand circles out; then circles in.

Using the above two movements, we now add arm motion. Circle your right arm and hand outward (once, slowly, like a long wave goodbye) following the direction of your body. Repeat three times, and then circle your arm and hand *inward*, following your body (slowly, four times).

4. Left hand circles out; then circles in.

Do the same exercise as above, only using your left hand this time. Four times each, in inward and outward circles.

5. Both hands circle out (Wave Hands Like Clouds).

Now bring both arms into it at once. Shifting your weight from side to side, circle your arms and hands *outward*, following your body. Four times.

6. Both hands circle in.

Both arms and hands circle *inward* as you are shifting weight from side to side.

7. Both hands circle to left.

Now circle both hands in the same direction, both turning counterclockwise. While you are shifting your weight to the left, circle your left arm and hand *outward* and your right arm and hand *inward*.

8. Both hands circle to right.

Now change directions, both hands turning clockwise. While you are shifting your weight to the right, circle your right arm and hand *outward* and your left arm and hand *inward*.

9. Left diagonal circle out, then circle in.

Step forward with your left foot to a forward lunge position. Shift weight forward and backward. At the same time, circle your left arm and hand forward (outward), following your body movement. After four times or more, change direction and begin to circle your left arm and hand backward (inward), following your body movement for the same number of repetitions.

10. Right diagonal circle out, then circle in.

Switch to a right foot, forward lunge position and do the same movement as above, shifting weight forward and backward. Circle your right arm and hand outward, smooth and slow, four or more times; then inward four or more times.

11. Left diagonal circle both hands

Return to the left forward lunge position (as in #9) and shift weight backwards and forwards, while circling both arms and hands outward smooth and slow, four times, and then inward four times.

12. *Right diagonal circle both hands.*

Move back into the right forward lunge position (as in #10). Shift weight forward and backward, both hands following your body movement in a circular motion, first outward four times; then inward four times.

13. *Brush (left) push (right).*

Move your left foot into a forward lunge position (as in #9). While you shift your weight back, circle your left arm inward; while you shift your weight forward, *push your right hand forward.*

14. *Brush (right) push (left).*

Step into a right forward lunge position (as in #10). While you shift your weight back, circle your right arm inward; while you shift your weight forward, *push your left hand forward.*

15. *Walking push hands.*

This is a tai chi movement; it is not easy to describe on paper because it is a multidimensional movement. You can get the DVD from our office if you need a visual demonstration.

Starting in a standing position, knees slightly bent, step forward into a small right forward lunge, while bringing arms up to chest height and pushing forward gently as you shift your weight forward slowly. Keep your hands and wrists soft, but determined.

As your weight shifts, bring left foot forward, pull hands back to solar plexus and push forward again, walking and pushing hands.

16. *Walking forward.*

We sometimes call this movement "Cat Walking" in tai chi practice. You walk with knees bent, landing on your heel and stepping down onto full foot in gentle steps. It is a well-controlled walk, and builds root energy.

17. *Walking backward.*

Same kind of walk as above, but now you land on your toe instead of heel as you move backward.

18. *Roll back arm (Repulse Monkey).*

As you walk backward, move your arm outward a half circle, then relax in an open position at shoulder-width, coordinating your arm motion with your body motion.

19. *Horse stance practice*

We discussed the horse stance previously. Step out with your left foot two times shoulder-width. Bend both knees and keep back relaxed and upright, pelvis tucked. Stay in this position for several minutes. Breathe.

— Tai Chi Qigong Exercise Sequence

I cannot stress this enough: Tai chi is qigong. It is a higher-level qigong. The sequence that follows is called tai chi movements in qigong practice. When you do it, you can really feel the energy flow in the body. Regular tai chi is practiced in a walking motion. But this form is practiced standing in one place. It is a lot easier than tai chi. I recommend the DVD from our office for your home practice.

1. *Preparation*

Feet at shoulder width apart. Relax whole body and mind, breathe deeply and quietly, mind focused on Dan Tian. Slowly raise your arms in front of body and inhale, then exhale lowering arms and sinking elbows, place hands in front of lower abdomen, and relax your lower back.

2. *Ward off*

Place left hand (palm facing downward) above right hand (palm facing upward), just like you are holding a ball. Move right hand to right side of body at shoulder level, place left hand next to left hip, shifting weight to right. Shift weight back to left placing hands to left like holding a ball on left with left hand above right hand. After repeating this 4 times, do the same movements on the opposite side: right hand (palm facing downward) above left hand (palm facing upward), just like you are holding a ball. Move left hand to the right side of body at shoulder level, place right hand next to right hip, shifting weight to left. Shift weight back to right, place hands to right like holding a ball on right with right hand above left hand. Do this 4 times. Breathe: inhale when holding ball, exhale when moving bottom hand out and when upper hand is next to hip.

3. Brush push

Shift weight to right side and push to right with left hand; then shift weight to left while circling right hand inward in front of body, left hand circles downward then outward until reaching shoulder level; then left hand pushes to right. Continue these movements 4 times, then do the same movement but on opposite side: shift weight to left side and push to left with right hand, then shift weight to right while circling left hand inward in front of body, right hand circles downward then outward until reaching shoulder level; push right hand to left. Repeat this movement 4 times. Breathe: inhale when circling hand inward, exhale when the other hand is pushing to the side.

4. Wind Blows Willow Tree

Shifting weight from left to right then from right to left; while at the same time, moving both arms and hands from left to right, then from right to left just following the body motion. Repeat this 4 times. Breathe: move hands to one side as you inhale, to the other side as you exhale.

5. Wave Hands

Circle left hand outward (to left) in the front of body as you shift weight to left; then circle right hand outward (to right) in the front of body as you shift weight to right, at the same time left hand on left side body gentle moves down. Repeat these movements 4 times. Breathe: wave to one side as you inhale, wave to the other side as you exhale.

6. Grasp Bird's Tail

This is a long continuous motion. Place left hand (palm facing down) above right hand (palm facing up), just like you are holding a ball (inhale). Move right hand to right side of body at shoulder level, place left hand next to left hip (exhale). Move left hand toward right hand (inhale), then shifting weight to left bring both hands downward the to the left (exhale, inhale); shifting weight to right while you move both hands to right in the front of your chest (exhale); shift weight to left moving both hands to Dan Tian area (inhale), then push to right (exhale). Do the same movements in the opposite direction: place right hand (palm facing down) above left hand (palm facing up), just like you are holding a ball. Move left hand to left side of body at shoulder level, place right hand next to left hip. Move right hand toward left hand; then shifting weight to right bring both hands downward the to the right; shift weight to left while you move both hands to left in the front of your chest; shift weight to right move both hands to Dan Tian area, then push to left.

7. *Ending*

Take three deep breaths as you gather energy from the universe, you can feel the energy moving through you body.

— **Sixteen Steps Tai Chi**

If you have practiced different forms of tai chi for a long time, you can start to do opposite mirror practice. This way will definitely enhance the brain benefits. The Sixteen steps tai chi form I created specifically for healing will enhance learning, and prevent brain aging. It took me a long time to create this form, not because I didn't know how, but because I needed to test this form with my students, and to have their feedback. I also needed to practice it to feel my own energy change. Many students told me, "This is the best I ever felt." It also took me a long time to find the right music to fit with this form. This is the form I used in my book, *tai chi for Depression*. The Sixteen Steps Tai Chi DVD can be purchased through our clinic. Find our contact information in the front of this book.

The characteristics of this tai chi form will give you an idea of what's involved:

- It is short, easy to learn, and easy to practice.
- Continuous circular movements create improved energy flow in the body.
- The martial arts characteristic empowers the mind, strengthens the body, and improves stamina and self-esteem.
- Symmetrical movements balance both sides of the brain to harmonize both brain activities and help you become well balanced.
- The sophisticated movements involve learning that stimulates brain cell communication and enhances your learning ability and creativity.
- The slow and balanced movements calm and balance the brain chemicals, increase serotonin level, reduce adrenalin level, and act as a natural tranquilizer.
- The moderate amount of physical movement enhances energy flow in the body and improves daily energy levels.
- The localized steps require a small space to practice, and can be practiced indoors when the weather is inclement.

- The coordinated, soothing, and open-frame movements (big frame) improve coordination and balance, open energy channels, and help you to open up to nature.

- Most movements are slow, soothing, calming, graceful, and peaceful; but there are some movements that are fast and powerful. It has yin and yang energies.

When you practice this form, you feel like you are empowered, more confident, strong, balanced, energy centered, and better able to control your life. You often feel better immediately after practice. This form can help you relieve the stress in your life and improve your daily energy level, immune function, and mental clarity. While you are learning tai chi, you're not just learning the exercise movements; you are actually learning about life and how to balance it.

Step Four: Cool-Down Movements

Whenever you exercise, you should always do some stretching and other cool-down movements afterward. It helps to support the relaxation of the muscles and joints, guarding against cramping and soreness. In addition, you will feel more relaxed and more open in your energy channels. An appropriate cool-down also helps to ensure that you get the most benefit possible from the exercise.

1. Reach up.

Inhale while raising one hand as high as you can, with your weight on the opposite foot. Exhale as lower your arm and hand and relax your body. Inhale again and raise your other hand as high as you can, with your weight on the opposite foot. Exhale as you relax your body and drop the arm and hand.

2. Stretching quadriceps.

Lift your left foot behind your buttock, and grab it with one or two hands, stretching your thigh muscle by pulling your foot gently closer to you buttock. Stretch for about one minute. Then change feet to stretch the other quad.

3. Stretching hamstring.

Move left foot in front of you with heel down and toe up. Bending forward with your left leg straight and your right leg bent. Try to grab your left toe (or just get as close as you can). Repeat on the right side. Then repeat on both sides again.

4. Forward bending, hands touching floor.

Take a deep breath and raise your hands above your head. Breathe out, bending forward slowly. Try to put your hands on the floor. Breathe and rest in that position for a count of ten seconds, before slowly bending back upright.

5. Forward lunge, stretching hip.

Take a long step forward with your left foot, bending at the knee; shift your weight to the front. Breathe and rest in that position for a minute or two. Change to the right foot and do the same thing.

6. Floor stretching.

Floor stretching can vary. You can use some yoga movements according to your own needs. I like the movements that twist the spine, with arms holding the knees.

7. Self massage on leg.

In a sitting position, you can easily massage your legs with your elbow.

8. Knee sitting (stretching Stomach Meridian).

This position is often seen in Japanese culture. It is really a "leg sitting" as you sit on both legs. This position is not only stretching the Stomach meridian, but also relaxes the lower back and allows the spinal fluid to flow more easily.

9. Self massage forehead, face, and neck.

Continue in the knee-sitting position, and massage your forehead for a minute; then massage your face for a minute; then massage your neck for a minute.

10. Ending with deep breathing and full relaxation.

Breathe slowly and deeply, put your awareness into each part of your body, making sure all of you is relaxed. If you still feel some tension, tense the area fully and quickly, and then release it, continuing to breathe through the tension, until you feel the full sensation of relaxation.

7
Where Am I On My Path?

We get distracted easily, by all different things. As we are just about to make a change, something else gets in the way. We often have excuses for not being able to do things for ourselves, especially things related to our health. We all know what to do, and how to do it. But we don't know how to be persistent. I too am often being distracted by so many things that are happening in my life. Fortunately, because of my tai chi and qi gong "habit," I can quickly catch up on things I am suppose to do for myself. I have taught many students over the past twenty years, and those who have been diligent about their learning, healing, and developing have made real changes in their lives.

Learning, healing, and developing the mind, the body, and the spirit takes time and effort. It requires dedication and determination. It is a lifestyle commitment. Furthermore, it is a smart move—you are embarking on a living revolution. If you ask yourself very often or consult your inner wisdom often enough, you already understand what is going on with you, and the answers to make things better are within you.

I had a patient who was going through some hard times and was under tremendous stress. She was trying to recover from health issues by seeing many different doctors, holistic practitioners, and even acupuncturists, but nothing seemed to work. She was upset, angry, confused, stressed, and tired of searching for answers in all different directions. She followed every instruction given by her doctors, therapists, and acupuncturists. She realized that all these medical professionals were saying different things, and this made her more confused. I finally had to ask her, "How much did you listen to *yourself?*"

She replied "Not at all."

I asked her, "Do you know what is really going on with your health?"

She said, "No, that is why I am going to all these practitioners and doctors!"

She had lost her common sense; she didn't even know what was going on in her own life and health. Her energy was totally chaotic and going in as many different directions as the number of things she was trying. Her brain network was tangled; the brain cells were not communicating with each other in efficient way. She could not breathe, suffocated by all this stress. Her confused mind could not make logical decisions for her healing path.

If this had been twenty years ago, I would have raised my voice and yelled, "Wake up, move, breathe, or get lost!" Instead, I gave her a big hug, and told her to follow her instincts to find out what are the things that are causing her stress. I guided her to let go of the thoughts that were troubling her. I provided treatment to her with affection and in a way that was natural, nurturing, and caring. I couldn't help but notice that I too had improved over the years—I think I was a little snobby twenty years ago, don't you?

We want to look at the course of our lives to see where our paths are leading. It doesn't matter if you are a left-brainer or a right-brainer, you can always make a difference. The difference is that you are always smarter than others about one thing: yourself.

I made this self-checklist for your convenience, but it's not necessary if you have already developed the of discipline self-awareness.

Self-Checklist

This is a self-assessment to find out where your practice has taken you. Rate your answers on a 1–5 scale, with the most positive being a five and the least positive a one. Don't put expectations on your score; when you've practiced for a long time, you may get a five. But if you get a low score, it is not necessarily a bad thing. It just means you need to practice more regularly and persistently. Nothing is impossible. Just open your mind to the possibilities. Think about doing this self-check once a month to know yourself better. Remember, as long as you put your mind to it, you will become what you are born to be and get everything you want.

1. Do I practice every day?
2. Am I focused when I am practicing these exercises?
3. Am I focused overall?
4. How is my balance overall?
5. How do I feel after each practice?

6. How was the tension in my body during practice?
7. How was the tension in my mind during practice?
8. How able have I been in dealing with stress?
9. How able have I been in social environments?
10. Is my memory getting better?
11. How is my learning ability?
12. How is my reading; is it faster than before?
13. Am I solving problems better?
14. How are my relationships with others?
15. Am I willing to explore more new things than before?
16. Am I able to do all the movements correctly?
17. How is my level of understanding of *qi*?
18. Do I feel the *qi*?
19. How is my confidence level?
20. What is my stress level?
21. What is my relaxation level?
22. How are my emotions when facing certain situations?
23. Am I calmer in general, better than before?
24. Am I more aware of my energy now, more than before?
25. Am I more willing to share my experience with others?
26. How is my mental creativity?
27. Do I have a goal now?
28. What is my goal now?
29. Am I generally stronger than before?
30. What is my fear level now, less than before?
31. What is my ultimate goal, will I reach it?
32. Do I agree with the following statements?

    - I am strong.

    - I can do anything I wish.

    - I can learn anything I wish.

    - I can heal myself.

    - I can change.

    - I am very confident about myself.

Final Note

Having lived in United States for twenty-one years, and having worked with many patients, including children, I have noticed that there is an urgent need: *natural health education should start at an early age*. I have seen so many children using medications, when they could instead be helped in a natural way. Children with weight problems, emotional problems, and other physical ailments can be helped with natural methods. Many adult problems come from childhood issues. Some people have had a poor lifestyle, some people have had an unhealthy diet, some took too many medications in childhood, or their focus on health was not a priority. I go to hospitals to visit my patients sometimes, and it is so crowded that I can hardly breathe. I then ask myself, *Why don't these people want preventive care?* The only answer I have is this: *They were never educated about natural medicine and healing.*

Here are a few suggestions that you should keep in mind:

- When your mind and emotions are stuck, move your body and participate in structured movement exercises.

- When you feel depressed or anxious, move your body and participate in structured movement exercises.

- When your healing is poor or not going anywhere, do body exercises.

- When you cannot use your mind anymore, use your body.

Here are a few things to remember.

- If you focus on disease, you have disease.

- If you focus on problems, you have problems.

- If you focus on life, you have life.

- If you focus on success, you will be successful.

- If you focus on the positive of everything, everything in your life will be positive.

A patient of mine asked me why we live, why are we in this world. I guess that he had suffered enough before this kind thought. I could not give an answer right way, because everyone has a different answer. And I won't give you one, but I am interested in yours. So I leave this to you, my reader. You can send me e-mail or post through Facebook, or write me a postcard to discuss this question.

We need to raise awareness of our health, our bodies and minds, our lifestyles, our healthful diets, and our movement options. We need to spread the word, telling people that there is a natural way for everything. We need to tell people, "Get up, move your body, and do something for your health."

We need to open our minds and see things from a wider angle, and not just in black-and-white. We need to accept things from both "traditional science" and "non-traditional science." We need to pay attention to our own bodies, our own energy, our own issues, our own behaviors, and stop putting the blame for our problems on others. We need to continue exploring, discovering, exercising, and of course, to never stop learning.

I wish you a great journey of exploring and learning.

Remember the Dao

Dao 63.3

    Deal with difficult things with simple acts.
    Deal with big things while they are small.
    Difficult tasks have easy beginnings.
    Large undertakings begin as small actions.

Dao 76.1

    At birth, a man is weak and flexible.
    At death, he is hard and rigid.
    All living things such as grass and trees,
    Are supple and yielding while alive,
    And withered and dry when they die.
    Thus unyielding rigidity is the companion of death,
    And yielding flexibility is the companion of life.

Dao 76.2

    Therefore an inflexible army will lose,
    The most rigid tree will snap.
    The hard and unyielding are lowered,
    While the soft and supple are elevated.

Dao 81:1

    Truthful words are not beautiful,
    Beautiful words are not true.
    The wise man is not learned,
    The learned man is not wise.
    The good are not many,
    The many are not good.

Dao 81:2

    The sage does not accumulate things.
    The more he does for others, the more he has.
    The more he gives to others, the more he receives.

Dao 81:3

> The Dao of heaven is to benefit without doing harm.
> The Dao of the sage is to act without contending.

Dao 67.2

> I have three treasures which I cherish and keep;
> The first is compassion,
> The second is frugality,
> The third is not daring to go first in the world.
> With compassion, one can be courageous.
> With frugality, one can be generous.
> With humility, one can be a leader of those who
> complete things.
> If one is courageous without compassion,
> If one is generous without frugality,
> If one takes the lead without humility,
> Then death is sure to follow.

Recommended Reading

Dennison, Paul E., and Gail E. Dennison. *Brain Gym and Me*. Ventura, CA: Edu-Kinesthetics, Inc., 2006. (Please visit http://www.braingym.org.).

Dyer, Wayne W. *Change Your Thoughts—Change Your Life: Living the Wisdom of the Tao*. Carlsbad, CA: Hay House, 2007.

Frantzis, Bruce. *Tai Chi: Health for Life*. Berkeley, CA: Blue Snake Books, 2006.

Formosa, Pamela. *Fraid Not: Empowering Kids with Learning Differences*. Bloomington, IN: iUniverse, 2009.

Katz, Lawrence C., PhD, and Manning Rubins. *Keep Your Brain Alive: 83 Neurobic Exercises*. New York: Workman Publishing Co., 1998.

Kuhn, Aihan, CMD. *Natural Healing with Qigong: Therapeutic Qigong*. Roslindale, MA: YMAA Publication Center, 2004.

———. *Simple Chinese Medicine: A Beginner's Guide to Natural Healing and Well-Being*. Roslindale, MA: YMAA Publication Center, 2009.

MacDonald, Matthew. *Your Brain: The Missing Manual*. Sebastopol, CA: Pogue Press, 2008.

Ratey, John J., MD. *A Users Guide to the Brain*. New York: Random House, 2002.

Wing, R. L., trans. *The Tao of Power: Lao Tzu's Classic Guide to Leadership, Influence, and Excellence* [A new translation of the Tao Te Ching]. New York: Doubleday, 1986.

Yang, Jwing-Min, PhD. *The Root of Chinese Qigong: Secrets for Health, Longevity, and Enlightenment*. Roslindale, MA: YMAA Publication Center, 1989, 1997.

Glossary

Bai Hui (Hundred Convergences): acupuncture point located at the top of the skull. The acupuncturist use this point to treat many ailments.

Brain Gym: describes a specific set of movements, processes, programs, materials, and educational philosophy. It is a registered trademark of the Educational Kinesiology Foundation (Brain Gym® International) in Ventura, California, USA.

Dao (Tao, Tao Te Ching): the way of nature, Classic text of Chinese philosophy. Written by Laozi, though its true authorship is still unresolved. The Tao Te Ching has had a great influence on all later schools of Chinese philosophy and religion and has been the subject of hundreds of commentaries.

Dan Tian: energy center in lower abdomen area

Jin: vital Essence stored in kidney

Meridian: Body energy pathway

Qi: Vital energy in the body

Shen: Vital spirit

TCM: Traditional Chinese Medicine uses various natural motholologies to assist healing,

Tui Na: Chinese massage involves many techniques and manipulation on the body to promotes Qi and blood circulation, remove stagnations and blockages in the body energy pathways.

Yin Yang: the concept of yin yang describes how contrary forces are interconnected and interdependent in the world, and how they support to each other..

Resources

Dr. Kuhn offers healing and learning retreat programs to help people to improve their skill in health, life and career. These programs include:

- The Secrets to Women's Health and Healing
- Answers for Better Relationships
- Brain Boot Camp
- Natural Healing for Post Traumatic Experience
- Things You Need to Know Before Getting Married
- Natural Methods for Relief from Anxiety
- Cancer Prevention Techniques
- The Road to Fearless Living
- The Secrets to Success
- Relieve Stress in Seven Minutes
- Unlocking the Secrets of Natural Medicine and Healing
- Medicine, East Meets West
- Lose Weight in Seven Days
- Cancer Healing Natural Way
- Qi Gong for Your Brain
- Emotion Healing through Body Movements

You can also bring Dr. Kuhn's programs to your facility.

Other Educational Programs:

- Qi Gong Instructor Training
- Tai Chi Instructor Training
- Wellness Tui Na (Theraputic Massage) Training

Books, DVDs, workshops, and appointments are available at
Chinese Medicine for Health, Inc.
1564A Washington Street
Holliston, MA 01746

To find out more or sign up for our newsletter,
please call us at (508) 429–3895
or visit www.ChineseMedicineforHealth.com

Books from Dr. Kuhn:

- Simple Chinese Medicine (Award-winning)
- Natural Healing with Qi Gong
- Tai Chi for Depression (sold only at Chinese Medicine for Health)

DVDs:

- Tai Chi Chuan (24 Steps, Yang Style)
- Tai Chi Chuan (42 Steps, Combined Style)
- Tai Chi Chuan (24 Steps, Chen Style)
- Tai Chi Sward (42 Steps, Combined Style)
- Tai Chi Fan (Single Fan)
- Tai Chi for Internal Healing (16 Steps)
- Therapeutic Qi Gong (36 Movements)
- Meridian Qi Gong
- Qi Gong for Arthritis
- Circle Energy Qi Gong
- Eight Brocade Qi Gong
- Twelve Minutes Qi Gong for Computer Users
- Tai Chi for Depression
- Dr. Kuhn Tai Chi Form Collection

Index

70
exercise, importance of, 59, 70
exercises
    for brain and memory, 100–106
    cool-down movements, 118–119
    for emotional balance, 106–111
    sixteen steps form, 117–118
    Tai Chi Qi Gong sequence,
        115–117
    warm-up exercises, 90–100

F
fear, 5
Feng Zhi Qiang, 17
fibromyalgia, 22, 55
financial planning, 37–38
forebrain, 30
forgetfulness. *See* memory
forgiveness, 76
friendships, 79

G
gastrointestinal benefits, 21–22
group energy, 12, 57–58

H
happiness, 70–79
hard work, 72–73
healing, 36–37
Healing and the Mind (Moyers), 3
health care system, 5
heart energy, 38, 69
helping others, 74
hindbrain, 30
hippocampus, 32–33
holistic medicine, 1
honesty, 73
Hundred Convergences, 87, 128

I
immune system, 23, 26
internal energy, 20
intuition, 75

J
Jet Lee, 17
jing, 9–10, 128

K
kidney energy, xiii, 9, 21, 29

L
learning, 43–44, 53, 59, 72–73,
    78–79
limbic system, 32
love, 79

M
Make the Most of Your Mind
    (Buzan), 39
mammalian brain, 32
meditation, 7, 12
memorization of numbers, 59
memory, 11–12, 28–29, 40, 42
mental training, 26
meridian system, 50, 128
midbrain, 30
mind processes, 70–72, 75–76
mind-body-spirit, 8–9, 12, 13
mindfulness, 61
Minding the Body, Mending the Mind
    (Borysenko), 3
Moyers, Bill, 3
musculoskeletal benefits, 22

music, 54, 60–61

Therapeutic Qi Gong, 22, 59